The New Experience
of Childbirth

Sheila Kitzinger is known and respected around the world as the leading authority on women's experiences of pregnancy, childbirth and motherhood. As a social anthropologist she has studied women's experiences of antenatal care, birth plans, midwifery, induction of labour, episiotomy, epidural anaesthesia and crying babies in many different countries. She lectures regularly in Europe, North and South America, Australia and Japan and her most recent books include PREGNANCY DAY BY DAY, BREASTFEEDING, THE NEW PREGNANCY & CHILDBIRTH, BIRTH YOUR WAY: CHOOSING BIRTH AT HOME OR IN A BIRTH CENTRE and REDISCOVERING BIRTH.

Sheila Kitzinger is married to Uwe Kitzinger and they have five daughters and three grandchildren.

The New Experience
of Childbirth

SHEILA KITZINGER

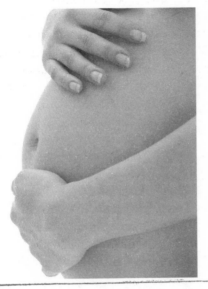

ORION

Photographs © Mother & Baby Picture Library/EMAP

This revised edition first published in Great Britain in 2004
by Orion,
an imprint of the Orion Publishing Group Ltd,
Orion House, 5 Upper St Martin's Lane,
London WC2H 9EA

A CIP catalogue record for this book
is available from the British Library.

ISBN: 0 75286 137 9

Typeset at The Spartan Press Ltd,
Lymington, Hants

Printed and bound in Great Britain by
Clays Ltd, St Ives plc

Contents

Acknowledgements

I want to thank my husband, Uwe, for his constant encouragement and understanding, and for helping to make my own
experiences of childbirth among the happiest memories of our
lives, and also our daughters – who have taught me feminism.
My special thanks to my daughter Tess, engineer and computer
wizard, who has had three home water births, and is an expert
communicator. I could not have produced this new version of
The Experience of Childbirth without her.

In the original edition of this book I expressed gratitude to
Baillière, Tindall and Cox for kindly allowing me to use six
illustrations from *Pictorial Midwifery* by Comyns Berkeley.
These are reproduced here on pages 161, 171, 172, 173, 174
and 175. The other sketches are by me. I realise that they are
amateur, but think of them as quick drawings I might do if I was
sitting beside you and I think they will make sense.

A Note to the Reader

This is not intended as a reference book. I have not added medical references because I did not want to intellectualise the birth experience. This book focuses on women's experience, not medical research. For those readers who want to look at the evidence I suggest that they read my book *The New Pregnancy & Childbirth* (Dorling Kindersley, 2003) and *Birth Your Way: Choosing Birth at Home or in a Birth Centre* (Dorling Kindersley, 2002). For the anthropology of birth and the history of medicalised birth, see my *Rediscovering Birth* (Little Brown, 2000).

The best source of information about the results of randomised controlled trials of different ways of caring for women in childbirth and obstetric interventions is the Cochrane Database. You will want the Pregnancy and Childbirth Database, and can access this at www.cochraneconsumer.com. The guide for Effective Care in Pregnancy and Childbirth tables is a good place to start exploring the website. It is divided into 'Beneficial Forms of Care', 'Forms of Care that are likely to be Beneficial', 'Forms of Care with a Trade-off between Beneficial and Adverse Effects', 'Forms of Care of Unknown Effectiveness', 'Forms of Care that are Unlikely to be Beneficial', and 'Forms of Care that are likely to be Ineffective or Harmful'.

Though randomised controlled trials are now accepted as the gold standard in research, there is a lot of other good research, some of which is qualitative. The Midwifery Information and Resource Service is another valuable source of information, with 6000 evidence-based references. This is on the website of the National Electronic Library for Health. Go to www.nelh. nhs.uk/maternity. The Informed Choice leaflets that you can read there include ones on 'Antenatal Screening', 'Place of Birth', 'Support in Labour', 'Fetal Heart Rate Monitoring', 'Ultrasound Screening', 'Alcohol and Pregnancy', 'Positions in Labour and Delivery', 'Breech Baby Presentation', 'Epidural Pain Relief' and 'Breastfeeding or Bottle Feeding'.

Following the birth of my first baby, and in the five years before the first edition of *The Experience of Childbirth* was published in 1962, I had been preparing women for childbirth with the National Childbirth Trust. During this time I had three more babies myself. (Then another one after it was published.)

Rereading my words in that edition I am astonished that the book could ever have been considered radical. But it was!

Those were the days when every woman who had babies was supposed to be married, and her main job was to support the male bread-winner. Self-confidence and social activism came very poor seconds to that.

The publication of *The Experience of Childbirth* was not only a sign of a developing self-assurance in women that challenged the medicalisation of birth, but also signalled a radical change in women's sense of themselves. The movement towards autonomy and choice and control in childbirth was a vital – though often neglected – element in the development of modern feminism. The birth movement was not just about making birth easier for individual women, but about the whole social and political context in which we give birth.

In this new edition I have added an introductory chapter, 'Birth: A Personal View', about birth in my life, setting birth activism in its social context and describing the changes that took place and the challenges we faced.

The sixties were the days when practices such as shaving the mother's perineum until it looked like a hard-boiled egg, administering massive doses of castor oil in an attempt to stimulate the uterus into action, insisting that the woman be bed-bound and forced to lie in a supine position throughout labour and birth, as well as routine episiotomy, were common and largely unquestioned. The term 'informed consent' had no meaning in childbirth. Women were supposed to be 'good patients' and do what they were told.

The first edition of this book was written pre-epidurals and before the Caesarean epidemic engulfed us. Twenty-five per cent of births in the USA are Caesareans. In the UK the rate is almost as high and still rising. This book came out before elective Caesareans were promoted as part of a spurious argument for women's rights, which appropriated feminist philosophy and incorporated it into obstetric marketing. It was before ultrasound was used to fix the estimated date of delivery – in fact a baby can be born two weeks before or after that date and be absolutely on time. It was before induction of labour with powerful drugs was seen as a solution to every pregnancy that went past term, and similar drugs were employed to rev up the uterus whenever labour was estimated as prolonged. And it appeared before the routine use of continuous electronic fetal monitoring and intravenous drips immobilised women and upped the Caesarean rate, without evidence that it saved babies' lives. In this edition I have included information about the benefits and risks of these interventions, and how a woman might cope with a 'managed' birth.

There have been advances. Today, clinical practice is intended to be evidence-based, at least in theory, and randomised controlled trials are considered essential to validate or to change practice. We have made some progress.

Yet for many women who give birth in a modern hospital where birth has been turned into a completely medical, or even a surgical, event, bringing new life into the world is an ordeal in which they are disempowered. They describe birth experiences in which they feel they have been violated. They use the language of rape. This is not merely a question of pain. For some pain was well controlled with drugs, but birth was still distressing and they are unhappy and panic-stricken afterwards because they felt utterly powerless. They relive the experience like a video on a loop that cannot be switched off. I created and run a Birth Crisis phone service for women who are suffering from post-traumatic stress after birth and need to talk about their experiences. You can contact this on (o)1865 300 266.

We shall only be able to humanise birth and reclaim it for women if we continue to ask searching questions, and have the

courage to challenge the obstetric management of a spontaneous physiological process and peak emotional experience in our
lives.

The quality of this experience depends not only on what is
taking place inside the pelvis, but on everything that is going on
in our minds. It is also profoundly affected by the relationships
we have with our care-givers, and by the interactions between
care-givers themselves. The purpose of this new edition of *The
Experience of Childbirth* is to empower women, and those who
serve them in childbirth, to understand and act on this.

Sheila Kitzinger
www.sheilakitzinger.com

A Note for Midwives

I am writing for midwives, too, but because I aim to stimulate reflection and personal insight into psychology and relationships, I cite few references to evidence-based trials in these pages, except where they are to do with emotions and birth experience.

I serve on the Midwives' Information and Resource Service editorial committee and suggest that midwives read the MIDIRS Midwifery Digest, which scans 500 journals, to keep up to date with information – www.midirs.org freephone 0800 581009.

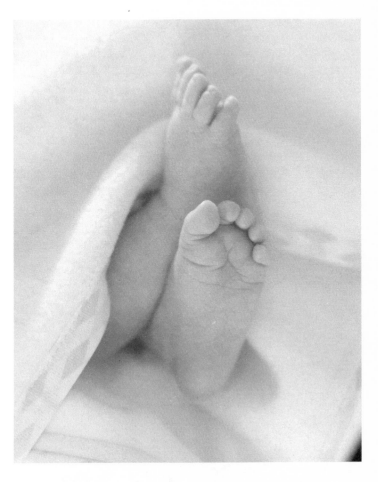

A pregnant woman does not know what her baby
will be like or how the birth experience will be. She is
on a journey of discovery.

I

Birth: A Personal View

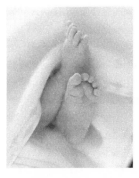

It never entered my head to hand over my body to doctors to deliver my baby. Uwe, my husband, was working with the Council of Europe and I was commuting between Strasbourg and Edinburgh University, where I was doing research and teaching in the Social Anthropology department. We knew our careers would lead us to work largely in different countries, and we both expected to be in control of our lives. Now I was pregnant. I had some direct experience of hospitals because in what would now be called a gap-year before university I had worked in one. I wanted none of the smells or sights or medical authoritarianism of hospital. I wanted to have my baby in my own way, at home, and to prepare myself so that I could experience birth with gusto.

I was lucky. I was healthy, happy and strongly supported by Uwe. I didn't for a moment expect a painless birth, but I knew I could cope, and just as you need skills to swim, or act, or to paint pictures – all things I enjoyed doing immensely – I believed that I could learn skills for childbirth. So I read everything I could lay my hands on, but I soon became critical of the kinds of training for childbirth that were available then. As I explored the physiological and emotional processes of giving birth – the mechanical breathing advocated by Fernand Lamaze, the entirely passive relaxation that Grantly Dick-Read disciples taught – I decided that I could invent skills myself.

Being in France gave me a cross-cultural view of birth. I compared and contrasted everything I learned about birth in Britain with how I saw friends having their babies within the small diplomatic community in Strasbourg. They had a choice between two nursing homes, and several highly regarded obstetricians. Each swore by one or the other. When I visited a friend who had just had her baby in the Catholic maternity home I saw that opposite her bed was a large crucifix, blood pouring from the gashes in Christ's side and down his legs, and from the thorn wounds in his brow. She said a crucifix had been right opposite her in the delivery room, too. The nuns were keen on breastfeeding. I watched how they made sure the baby was 'on'. The nun stood at the door, with the baby tightly bundled in her arms like one of the pink or blue sugared almonds that were the conventional gift to a new mother, shouted, 'Brace yourself, mother!', and ran at her with the baby, whose mouth was wide open with shock, and latched the infant firmly on the breast. The other maternity home was a little more liberal. But I did not intend to be managed, one way or the other. I firmly believed that women had the ability to give birth and to breastfeed their babies. They should not be treated as compliant children or complete idiots.

Of course, my interest in childbirth began long before that. My mother had been a midwife. I'd pored over her midwifery books with fascination as a child and she had influenced me greatly. In Taunton where we lived, she started one of the first Family Planning clinics in the south west of England, collaborating with my Aunt Liz in Devon, a virago of a woman who was a radical socialist and passionate about social causes. For the first time, effective contraception was made available free of charge to women of all social classes. The poor could start to have some control over their own lives. I remember going from school to meet my mother at the clinic and seeing shabby, down-trodden women slipping out of the doors, flustered, pleased, proud, with mysterious packages, clutching them like Christmas presents. I heard her talking about the ethics of her work, her reasons for doing it, the day-to-day experiences of counselling, and the stories she heard of male violence, extreme poverty and distress. No girl could grow up and not be influenced by that.

That was one of the strands which led to my choice of university course. It was to be either psychology or social anthropology. In the end it was social anthropology at Oxford. My supervisor of studies, John Peristiany, was a remarkable man. Instead of making me toe the line, he encouraged creativity, constant questioning and the application of all that I was learning academically to everyday life. He felt himself marginal to Oxford. He had not been to the same schools as most other dons, was not part of the old boy network, so perhaps that was why he was able to think laterally. The education I received as an undergraduate reinforced my determination to challenge orthodoxy, wherever I became aware of its flaws – and that applied nowhere more than in the care given to women in pregnancy and childbirth.

Astonishingly, though, while I was at Oxford I learned hardly anything about women's lives in different cultures. Women were invisible. Social anthropology at that time was all about men: political and economic systems, the ways men controlled inheritance, the rites by which they became warriors. Professor Evans-Pritchard was a specialist in the Nuer of the Southern Sudan. There were more references to cows in the indices of his books than there were to women. Yet it was obvious that women kept the whole system going. Without them men would not have been fed and nurtured. They would have been starving and homeless. Without them children would not have survived. Women were being used as pawns to exchange in a complicated exhibition of male power.

The important experiences of women's lives were hidden and largely unrecorded, except by a handful of female anthropologists – Ruth Benedict and Margaret Mead among them – who examined motherhood and childrearing. Margaret Mead came to Oxford and conducted seminars for us at the Institute of Social Anthropology. When I told her I was unhappy with the content of the Oxford anthropology course she encouraged me to explore further.

The first opportunity for fieldwork came when I got to know a group of prostitutes who catered for American airmen at a base outside Oxford. Taxi drivers in Gloucester Green ran a flourishing business transporting Americans into Oxford, introducing them to these women, and letting them use their taxis for quick sex. The women were mostly girls who had run away because they were unhappy at home. Some of them had been sexually abused by men in the family. They talked to me frankly and I listened and learned. I told John Peristiany about this. He was the kind of person you could talk to about such subjects and he urged me to use my anthropology to organise and analyse the information I was getting. My first piece of what was virtually field research is remembered with some horror by now elderly dons.

For my thesis I did more formal research into the lives of African, West Indian and Asian students in British universities, and developed interview techniques and skills in participant observation. Mainly, I learned how to listen and how to record in detail even things that seemed insignificant at the time. As a result of reading social anthropology, from the beginning of my research into pregnancy and birth I looked at cultures comparatively, and many friendships grew out of the work. Oxford was for me a multi-cultural experience.

So it was inevitable that when I became pregnant I brought with me both the passion of my mother's practical feminism and everything I had gleaned about women's lives in other cultures, to make my birth experience what I wanted it to be, to challenge the medical model of birth, and to be assertive and confident.

My first baby was born at home in France, with a midwife and Uwe present. In the middle of labour I suddenly felt, 'This is a sport I can do!' At school I had never been any good at gym or games. Now I found my body functioning perfectly. Labour lasted two and a half hours. I crouched grasping the bulbous leg of a Victorian table that I had restored and painted with black and yellow stripes like a bee, and then, because the midwife asked me to, got on the bed to push the baby out. It was a perfect birth, except that I tore. I needed stitching up. That was because, as the midwife agreed, she had been nervous about this birth, and had ordered me to push before I had had the irresistible urge. I was carted off to one of the maternity homes to be sutured and there was a bumpy ride back in an ambulance. I walked in the Black Forest later that week to work the uncomfortable stitches loose. All was well. Though the wound hurt, my GP in Oxfordshire told me eight weeks later she would never have known that my perineum had been sutured. This was the beginning of my special interest in the way the second stage is conducted and the genital mutilation that is often inflicted on women in our culture.

I was fortunate that breastfeeding went beautifully, and I never considered giving the baby a bottle although she did not gain much weight. We returned to Oxford six weeks after Celia's birth. Mother met me on the steps of the Randolph hotel. Her first comment was, 'Oh, she's very small.' I had produced an inadequate offering. Then I was in trouble with the health visitor. 'What are you feeding her?' she asked. I said breastmilk. 'Aren't you giving her anything else?' When I replied that I was not, and in response to subsequent questioning added that I was a vegetarian, the health visitor was horrified. 'You need to give her mashed brains. If you don't give her any brains she won't develop any.'

Soon after Celia arrived, I started voluntary work with the National Childbirth Trust and, in the sixties, was the first to begin couples' classes and counselling for couples before and after childbirth. Later on, in the seventies, with an NCT colleague, I created the teacher training scheme, based on the tutorial system.

My second pregnancy turned out to be twins, and Tess and Nell were born at home too, before Celia was two years old. I had reserved a hospital bed but prepared for everything at home. It was just as well, since one baby was born an hour and a half after the first signs of labour, and the other ten minutes later. If I had attempted to go to hospital when labour hotted up they would probably have been born in a lay-by on the Oxford by-pass.

After my third home birth – a torrential, painful, but glorious forty minutes of action – a couple of years later, I started to write my first book, *The Experience of Childbirth*. Polly was waking for a feed around five in the morning, and I used the quiet time for writing as silvery light spread through the sky. I submitted the manuscript to Victor Gollancz, known for his progressiveness. I included a few photographs taken by Uwe of me giving birth, breathing my way through contractions, smiling as I reached down to stroke a glistening head that had just emerged, and cradling a naked baby against my breasts. My brother-in-law, Hilary Rubinstein, worked at Gollancz then. Victor called him into his office and announced, apparently with shocked disbelief, 'I have photographs of your sister-in-law's private parts on my desk.' The manuscript was accepted immediately, just as it stood. Its publication, and serialisation in a Sunday paper, brought a tide of letters from women sharing their experiences, many of whom seemed to find a voice for the first time. That was the start of a stream of letters, stories, poems, phone calls and, as time went on, emails, from women around the world. It was as if I had pulled out a cork so that wine could flow. Women poured out their joy and anguish, their anger and their love, describing their births and telling me how hospitals, doctors and midwives needed to change.

The language to convey the powerful physical sensations and overwhelming emotions of birth had to be created. Women had been silent because there was no way in which to express their feelings. Birth was discussed only as 'pain', as if that were the sum of what labour and birth were about. Opening your body to let new life into the world is much more than that and has always had multiple layers of meaning for a woman, and for everyone else involved.

My last baby was born two years after Polly, also at home. It was a longer labour, took five hours, and consisted mostly of backache, but this time it was without a midwife. I was waiting for contractions to feel more effective and, when suddenly a storm of pushing sensations swept through me, we were not quick enough to get one. Uwe filmed and said, 'Smile, darling!' while the baby crept out by herself and then up to my breast.

Jenny was two when the whole family went to Jamaica, where for nine months I did research on the experiences of birth and motherhood for women who lived in Lawrence Tavern, and in Trenchtown and on the Dunghill in Kingston (a massive rubbish dump where people live in makeshift shacks and the shells of old cars).

I had a base with the Medical Research Council on the university campus, but my days were spent in women's homes up in the hills and in the poorest parts of the city. At the Victoria Jubilee Hospital I saw the degrading and brutal treatment of women in childbirth in an institution in which a superficial veneer of modern medicine mixed with desperate attempts at crowd control and the vitality of Jamaican culture to produce a scene like a Bosch painting of purgatory. There was a pillow in each of the delivery rooms. I only ever saw it used for pressing over the face of a screaming woman to silence her. Drugs for pain relief were available only with operative or assisted deliveries, and there was no other help with handling pain. Women tried to get upright, to move, to rock and roll their pelvises, to crouch and to kneel. But their efforts were considered primitive behaviour by midwives, mainly trained in Britain and Canada, and the mothers were goaded up on to hard, narrow delivery tables, if they could make it in time, to be routinely delivered flat on their backs. They often had to share beds, too, one at the head end, another at the foot. Membranes ruptured and blood leaked from one woman into the genital tract of the other. Faeces, urine, amniotic fluid, blood all mixed. The women clutched each other and rocked, groaned, sang verses of the Psalms. The only thing I could do was to say, 'I have had five children', and to try to share the experience with them. I tried to offer them firm physical support so that they could move freely, and often I climbed up on the delivery table and cradled them in my arms to give birth. Midwives were worked off their feet. If I was with a woman giving birth they tended to leave me alone with her so I was able to be woman-to-woman. Then the screaming would stop. Instead women rocked, breathed, moaned and sang. I learned that these women could, without any birth classes, give birth beautifully, rhythmically, joyfully.

Jamaica was the first country where I was able to observe childbirth in women, exactly like me, yet who came from a completely different culture, who often could not read or write, and I learned that all over the world women shared the intense experience of birth in similar ways, and that we had the innate and expert skills to give birth perfectly.

It was that direct experience of the vital importance of woman-to-woman companionship in birth that sharpened my insight so that I came to understand the long tradition of female help and empathy in all cultures, and throughout European history. Women have always been together during childbirth. To isolate them from each other and cut them off from their own inner feelings, to force women to get on a bed and lie still, to subject them to management, however kindly, fixes birth in a medical straitjacket. It obstructs the physiological process and increases the need for other medical and surgical interventions. In the process birth is made more traumatic and often dangerous. Every obstetric and midwifery intervention – even apparently minor ones like breaking the waters or getting a woman up on a bed – introduces the need for further interventions: induction of labour leads to strong painkilling drugs, further artificial uterine stimulation, more drugs, assisted delivery or Caesarean section, possible haemorrhage and infection, a baby who has to be admitted to the intensive care nursery, and to postnatal physical illness, depression or post-traumatic stress disorder, inability to breastfeed, and so on.

My personal experiences have been the sparks that fire my enthusiasm to help other women have births as exultant as mine and to be there for them when they have traumatic experiences that they need to talk through. This includes being there for women prisoners and asylum seekers.

Today, every woman who has her baby in hospital is turned into a patient. She becomes a temporary member of a tightly organised, hierarchic and bureaucratic medical system. The admission procedure marks the point at which the institution takes control of her body. It is a ceremony in which she is registered, classified, examined, the fetal heart rate is recorded, and her blood pressure measured.

In most hospitals you have to surrender your own clothing, a symbol of individuality. You may be separated from friends and family, with the exception of a designated birth partner. You are expected to be like a child, to follow instructions, avoid drawing attention to yourself, and behave nicely. You may be addressed by your first name, but will not call the obstetrician by his or her first name. Or you may lose your name altogether, and be referred to by professionals as 'the Caesarean in Room 16', 'the pre-eclampsia case', 'the grand multip', 'the induction'.

When interns in a Boston hospital were asked to define a 'good patient', one doctor answered, 'She does what I say, hears what I say, believes what I say . . .'[1] A good patient is compliant. She thanks the professionals because they 'save' her baby. She is grateful regardless of what they do to her. If she fails to conform she is seen as a 'difficult patient'.

Birth is regulated by artificial hormones and often completed by surgery. A woman may be tethered to electronic equipment, numbed by anaesthesia from the waist down, and have her uterus artificially stimulated. Then an episiotomy is performed and she is delivered by forceps or vacuum extraction. The doctors may decide on a Caesarean section. On the other hand, they may think it better to avoid labour entirely, and schedule an elective Caesarean. Some women actually ask for one, because they have been led to believe that it is the easiest, safest and most pain-free way to have a baby.

When I studied social anthropology I realised that we can look at the social system of the hospital as if it were a society in Africa or anywhere else in the world. A hospital has protocols that make for easy management, so that those at a higher level can regulate the actions of their subordinates. Routines ensure that people co-operate in tasks without asking awkward questions or having to think. They are rarely challenged. When research is published that shows things done to women

---

[1] Scully, D., *Men Who Control Women's Health*, Houghton Mifflin, Boston, 1980.

in childbirth are useless or harmful, it takes around fifteen years for obstetric practice to change.[2]

Birth is treated as a medical event which not only usually takes place in hospital but is thought about almost exclusively in terms of risks. If you decide to give birth at home you may have to overcome many obstacles put in place by the medical system. Family members and friends say, 'You're very brave!', 'Aren't you worried that something will go wrong?', 'You are being selfish' or 'You're not thinking about the baby'.

A woman who wants to give birth as naturally as possible and have no drugs, and who chooses midwife care, may be transferred to specialised obstetric management as soon as there are any signs that her labour does not conform to a standard. Midwives are often anxious about the responsibility they take on when they attend out-of-hospital births – even births in 'home-from-home' rooms in the hospital. So a woman who hopes to give birth without interventions is wheeled across the corridor or transported by ambulance to high-tech care, often simply because her membranes ruptured early or labour is slow.

A normal labour in a healthy woman tends to be treated with all the interventions that are characteristic of high-risk labours. Because birth is treated as high-risk, it often *becomes* high-risk.

Everything I have learned in my work from women in other cultures and around the world has convinced me that our med-icalised way of birth is not the only way, and not, for the majority of women, the best way. We need to learn from each other. Yes, there are high-risk pregnancies and births where we should be grateful for the support of obstetric skills and high-tech intervention. But for most of us these complicate and impede the normal physiological process, make birth traumatic, and often leave women emotionally mutilated.

I am privileged to be part of a great international movement to reclaim childbirth for women and for families. It started almost apologetically in the sixties. We asked whether women

---

[2] Lomas, M., Enkin, M., et al, 'Opinion leaders vs audit and feedback to implement practice guidelines', *Journal of American Medical Association* 265, 1991, pp. 2202-7.

in childbirth could be treated as human beings, might be consulted about what was done to them, could learn ahead of time what was likely to happen and how they might be treated, and how they could prepare themselves with relaxation and breathing.

In the seventies and eighties this approach changed to become open criticism of medical power and a demand for full information and a right to share in decision-making. In 1982 the Professor of Obstetrics at a major London teaching hospital issued an edict that women could not labour and give birth off the bed, and that they must lie back against pillows instead of standing, kneeling, squatting or being on all fours. So Janet Balaskas, founder of the Active Birth Movement, and I decided to organise what we thought was going to be a small demonstration outside the hospital. My phone rang the night before and a voice announced itself as the Director of Crowd Control for Scotland Yard. He told me that we were going to have so many supporters that we must switch the demonstration to Parliament Hill Fields and that mounted police would be out to help us. There were going to be so many people that, though we could start to congregate in front of the hospital, there would be no space for everyone, and we must march. The next day we had five thousand people out on the street. The Professor resigned, and from then on women could give birth in any position they liked, on or off the bed.

In the nineties came the rebirth of midwifery in countries, like the USA and Canada, where it had been virtually destroyed, and a reassertion, at first timid but later more confident, of the autonomy of midwives in countries such as Britain and New Zealand, and increasingly in other European nations. This came about because of demands by women, decisive action and good publicity. I remember how with midwives and mothers in Ontario I marched in front of the Medical College to call for the legalisation of midwifery. The police told us that we had to keep moving. That was fine by me. So I led the march with my life-like baby doll and home-made foam rubber vagina, birthing a baby, and rocking and rolling my pelvis in a birth dance, along the street, with the TV cameras rolling.

Protest about the dehumanisation of childbirth always needs to be informed by research and by carefully listening to women across the world. I have studied, lectured and learned from women in countries as far apart as South Africa, the Caribbean, Japan, Australia, Colombia, Mexico, Hungary, Iceland and Russia, as well as in almost all the countries of Europe, and around North America. It is exhilarating. Women are starting to speak out.

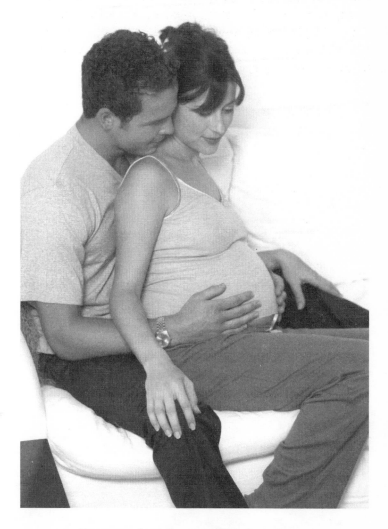

Pregnancy is not just a waiting time. It is an opportunity for emotional growing and for a couple to understand each other with greater sensitivity.

2

Childbirth with Joy

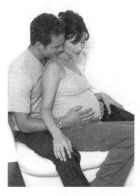

The experience of bearing a child is often central to a woman's life. Years after the baby has been born the mother remembers acutely the details of her labour and her feelings as her baby slipped out of her body. Speak to any grandmother about birth and almost immediately she will begin to talk about her own labours. It is unlikely that any experience in a man's life is comparably vivid.

When women have suffered in childbirth – have felt humiliated and degraded by being the passive instruments of interventions they could not understand and to which they did not give their fully informed consent – it is not only they who are affected. They carry with them through their lives the memory of this experience, and by their attitude towards child-bearing affect other women and men – not only their own daughters and sons, but many others with whom they come into contact.

Childbirth is not a curse laid on Eve, a path of suffering to be trod so as to have the joy of children. It can be an exciting challenge, rewarding in itself, and not simply a means to an end.

The way a woman feels about pregnancy and birth, and her whole manner of approaching it, are aspects of her sense of herself as a woman – and part of her sexuality. Sex is not just something that happens in our genitals. A woman's psychosexual life encompasses pregnancy, birth, giving herself to the baby physically as well as emotionally, feeding and touching it, and also includes the way she feels and thinks about her body in relation to other people's bodies. It is difficult for a man to understand – hard, too, for any woman who has had an average hospital birth – how birth can be sexual. But it can be one of the most profound psychosexual experiences in a woman's life. Each contraction may bring a rush of joy so overwhelming that pain recedes into the background because in an intense psychosexual experience there is a surge of endorphins. These are hormones released into the bloodstream during energetic activity. They are natural painkillers which produce a 'high' rather like that felt by athletes when they are pouring all their energy into strenuous and satisfying physical activity. In the second stage of labour the pressure of the baby's head against the walls of the vagina and the fanning out of tissues as the head descends also brings for some women an unexpected sensation of sexual arousal, and even of ecstasy. I do not claim that birth is orgasmic, but it is joyous – and can be blissful.

I remember a scene in my grandmother's house when I was about seven. The aunts and grown-up cousins were in the sitting room, and as I passed the seed-cake politely from one to the other I heard cousin Gladys whisper to my mother that cousin Rose was expecting a baby. The conspiracy of women over the tea-cups and the hushed tones in which the information was conveyed told me that this was special and rather shocking news. Later that day I shared my precious secret with another, younger, cousin. She was disbelieving. I cannot remember whether it was because Rose was not married, or whether she did not have a gooseberry bush, or the stork had not visited. But she asked, 'How can they *know*?' and, having pored over my mother's midwifery books, unfortunately I told her. I got into dreadful trouble about it and was obviously considered a contaminating influence. I felt unclean for a long time after. And I do not remember that carefully brought up little cousin ever being left alone with me again.

This was not in the Dark Ages (though it makes me feel part of history), but the casual way in which I can now tell the story contrasts strongly with the crimson rush of shame I felt on being found out. I should like to think that Rose enjoyed giving birth to her baby, though I doubt she did. Anyway, she obviously stayed in the back of my mind, and the sense of outrage and injustice I felt on her behalf spurred me into doing something to help women give birth with awareness, understanding and delight.

I hope that the way many women still feel about childbirth – with a sense of dread, wanting to hand over their bodies to professionals, not feel anything, and get it over with as quickly as possible – that before my grandchildren have babies, all this will look as out of date as the story about Rose.

PAIN

Pain in labour is real enough. We dare not underestimate the agony that some women endure in childbirth. It is not to be lightly glossed over by those more fortunate. Whether or not childbirth, as a natural function of the female body, *should* be easy, it cannot be denied that for a great many women it is not. One woman described to me how, commanded to push as long, energetically and as often as she possibly could, she gritted her teeth so hard during the second stage that she chipped off a front tooth. Labour can be one of the most painful experiences a human being can suffer. Pain 'as measured by the thermal radiation method is reported in some women to reach 10 to 10½ dols'.[1] 'This degree of pain is the most extreme pain that human beings are capable of feeling and is comparable to the pain felt in extreme forms of physical torture or third-degree burns.'[2] It can hardly be expected that a woman who goes

---

[1] C. T. Javert and J. D. Hardy, 'Measurement of pain intensity in labor and its physiologic, neurologic and pharmacologic implications', *Am. J. Obst. and Gynae.*, 60: 522, 1950.
[2] Niles Newton, *Maternal Emotions*, Hoeber, USA, 1955.

through that sort of experience should feel positive about child-bearing or can help a pregnant woman feel joyful anticipation of the great adventure that confronts her.

Women *feel* pain differently; and this is probably affected as much by social factors as by sheer physiology or by anything which might be uncovered by psychoanalytic techniques. Pain is always interpreted and placed within a predetermined context. When I was doing anthropological research in Jamaica I discovered that the West Indian peasant woman rarely feels discomfort on the perineum, or minds the pressure of the baby's head as it descends. But the English middle-class woman worries about dirtying the bed and is often shocked by sensations against the rectum and the vagina in labour – sensations which she may find excruciating. She feels distressed, in fact, at just those sensations which the peasant woman meets with equanimity.

On the other hand a Jamaican peasant woman often anticipates and gets severe backache, a common enough experience all over the world. To her this pain is evidence of the back 'opening up' – which she believes it must do before the child can be born. Cross-cultural and other sociological factors must be considered if we really want to understand what childbirth is all about.

There is more to birth than pain. Pain is often turned into suffering because of the way in which a woman is treated by those caring for her. She could handle straightforward pain, but medicalised birth makes her feel trapped and helpless. A woman may have a labour in which pain is eradicated by epidural anaesthesia and yet still come out of it feeling degraded and cheated. Birth doesn't have to be like that. When a woman has her baby happily she spreads a different spirit – a mood of gladness.

It is this joy in birth that can be the essence of childbirth – birth in which a woman finds delight in the rhythmic harmony of her body's functioning. Without this spirit, attaining perfect mechanical action in labour is not only made more difficult, but, even if achieved, is strangely unsatisfying.

Nowadays there is no reason why birth should entail suffering, with or without preparation. But the concern of this book is with a more positive experience. It is childbirth with joy.

Bodies are for feeling with, and for actively living through and enjoying. When the healthy body is engaged in a natural physiological process an individual normally feels pleasure and content. We enjoy eating and drinking and defecating, settling down to sleep and waking refreshed, walking, jogging and swimming, breathing the sea air, and making love. In repose and activity, in relaxation and effort, harmonious and co-ordinated physical function brings sensations of well-being. It can be the same with childbirth.

I do not claim that if a woman thinks about birth in the way I describe, and does breathing and relaxation exercises, she is bound to have an easy labour. What I hope to do is help her see a pattern and meaning in childbirth, and to understand it not as something that is done *to* her, but as a profound psychosexual experience.

Giving birth is not a matter of success or failure, or of putting on a splendid performance, but of giving yourself, mind and body, to a creative experience in which, literally, love is made flesh.

'NATURAL BIRTH'

The history of the 'natural childbirth' movement has been one of unfortunate, though perhaps inevitable, conflict – not only between those who believed in its value and others who felt that it was all pointless, but between exponents of different theories. It is probably a mistake to look for a single evolution of ideas and methods. There has been spontaneous and independent development in different countries over the last fifty years.

The Pioneers

Concern over women's emotional adjustment to childbirth was first expressed by Grantly Dick-Read in the thirties. His books formed the basis of preparation for childbirth in Britain today. Other important factors in the natural childbirth movement were advances in obstetric physiotherapy stemming largely from the work of Helen Heardman, which in its turn owed a lot to physiotherapist Kathleen Vaughan, who learned from traditional Indian ways of birth, and to another physiotherapist, Minnie Randall.

In France the psychoprophylactic method (*accouchement sans douleur* – ASD) is associated with the name of Fernand Lamaze, a French obstetrician working in a Communist trade clinic in a grimy *quartier* of Paris. On a visit to the Soviet Union he was impressed by the calm in maternity wards practising this method. He brought the theories behind this method back with him to Western Europe, and invented new techniques – notably the 'panting like a dog' method of riding over contractions. ASD owed its origins to Pavlovian psychology (the same Pavlov who did research on salivating dogs) and antenatal training used in Soviet hospitals. Lamaze in turn was followed by Pierre Vellay, who had a very elegant private maternity clinic in Paris where a footman served champagne on a silver salver to newly delivered mothers. The exponents of these theories read their Dick-Read too. But they claimed their approach was different in that it was based on building a series of conditioned reflexes which raised the pain threshold, so that sensations formerly interpreted by the brain as painful were accepted as painless.

These techniques coming largely from France and Russia (and also widely practised in China) aim to eliminate painful sensations but, to the cost of some women who adopted them, neglected that exhilaration which comes in childbirth in which a woman actively participates, when pain may exist in the background but is brushed aside as being not nearly so important as the business of having a baby, or is willingly experienced as something which can be controlled.

Women who imagined that their labours would be completely painless often suffered an unpleasant shock, and if not prepared for the powerful sensations and astonishing force of uterine contractions may have panicked and been worse off than if they had not been to classes at all.

A problem with psychoprophylaxis (literally 'mind prevention') was that it treated birth as if it were an exam which a woman either passed or failed. When Fernand Lamaze reported his results at his Paris clinic he announced that over 18 per cent of women succeeded completely, but just over 4 per cent 'failed'. He did not mean by this that they did not have a baby. They lost control and were restless or screamed. They had failed in 'the method'.

We have a very grave responsibility if a woman is trained for childbirth only to feel that she must put on a star performance and that she has failed at the first real pain.

Most women must expect pain or great discomfort at the end of the first stage. If pain is great a woman should be able to choose to have drugs to kill it, or at least take the edge off contractions, and pain-relieving drugs should always be available.

But all analgesics and anaesthetics bring with them risks for the baby. Few mothers are able to look back on their labours and say, as Queen Elizabeth said when she opened a building of the Royal College of Obstetricians and Gynaecologists, 'You have given almost literal meaning to Wordsworth's assertion that "Our birth is but a sleep and a forgetting." '[3] Moreover, many women, far from welcoming the opportunity, do not like the idea of facing the most important moments of their lives either unconscious or unable to feel anything at all. It is for this reason rather than because of the risks of anaesthesia that Dr Guttmacher's account of childbirth in the USA in the 1950s, the days of 'twilight sleep',[4] seems to me to make sad reading:

> In favourable cases, under the influence of the drug triad, the patient falls into a deep quiet sleep between pains, but groans and moves about in a restless manner with each pain. The somnolent state continues into the second stage of labour and frequently for several hours after delivery. When the patient awakes, the obstetrician is rewarded by hearing her

---

[3] As reported in the *Guardian*, July 16th, 1960.
[4] *Having a Baby*, Signet, USA, 1950.

ask, 'Doctor, when am I going to have my baby?' The quickest way I know to prove that the child is already born is to have her feel her own abdomen. A newly restored waist-line soon convinces even the most sceptical.

Although you can show a woman how to have a baby just as she might learn how to make a soufflé, the whole thing may fall pretty flat at the last moment. Childbirth is not – and never has been – sheer obstetric dexterity and several thousand pounds to the magician who is doing it all for you. Nor is it an intellectual exercise for which you sit through a course soaking up academic information; after all, a great many women who don't know their pelvis from their perineum have borne their babies easily and with all the thrill of achievement. Nor is it an athletic performance for which one needs muscles like a boxer's biceps or an abdominal wall like the kitchen table. Nor simply a matter of squatting down amongst the leaves with the squirrels and little wild creatures and having it 'naturally'; today's obstetric skills are too precious for both the mother and the baby to forgo for that particular chimera. Joy in childbirth is a matter of the woman's expectations about labour, her relations with her body and her feelings about child-bearing, her deepest hopes and fears, her relationship with her partner and her parents, her acceptance of a new role, and the way in which she co-ordinates all these emotions and relationships. Then even physical difficulties can frequently be surmounted and fall into the background within the total picture of psychosomatic harmony.

A Woman's Active Role

It is not the absence of pain that gives value to the approach suggested in this book, but the addition of qualities which can make birth a thrilling adventure and a revelation which a couple can share. In this sense childbirth can be an experience through which we grow to greater spiritual and psychological fullness.

A woman is no longer a passive, suffering instrument. She does not hand over her body to doctors and midwives to deal with as they think best. She retains the power of self-direction, and makes choices between alternatives. That may include the decision to turn to obstetric skills for help. For every labour is different and the most that a woman can do is to handle her labour in the best possible way for her. To do this effectively she needs knowledge of the processes of pregnancy and birth, and a mind which is not only free of all fear but filled with pleasurable anticipation. To achieve rhythmic co-ordination and harmony she must, above all, *trust her body and her instincts*.

You cannot stumble into this sort of childbirth without preparation. Quite often women have quick or easy labours, but even these do not bring the fullness of joy – the birth passion – which comes from a labour in which a woman, despite pain, is utterly triumphant.

The end result of preparation for birth is not athletic skill, super-elastic muscles or the ability to breathe like a Yogi or relax until you are in a hypnotic stupor, but a mental state: self-confidence and an emotional preparedness without which no amount of physical exercise is adequate preparation for the experience of labour.

Emotional preparedness was the basis of Grantly Dick-Read's emphasis on fearlessness and the clearing away of psychological obstructions so that a woman could have her baby as nature intended. We cannot afford to lose the spirit that shone through Dick-Read's courageous work in the early days when the whole subject seemed suspect to many leaders of the medical profession.

I am aware that there are people who find all mystical notions about childbirth unacceptable, and certain of Dick-Read's most sincerely felt statements of a metaphysical kind brought him into disrepute with some who prided themselves on their practical natures. I would not suggest that we should approach childbirth borne on the wings of a pseudo-mysticism which might collapse at the crucial moment. Nevertheless, to anyone who thinks about it long enough, birth cannot simply be a matter of techniques for getting a baby out of your body. It involves our relationship to life as a whole, the part we play in the order of things; and, as the baby develops and can be felt moving inside, to some women annunciation, incarnation, seem to become facts of their own existence.

Physical preparation is, however, important and relaxation forms its basis, the prerequisite without which a happy labour is unlikely. And yet there is a good deal of misunderstanding as to what this relaxation really means.

Childbirth with joy does not mean that a woman, having learned to relax as if on a sunny seashore, basking in delicious warmth, just lies down whilst her labour proceeds without her, and does not feel contractions or notice what is happening to her. In many hospitals and clinics relaxation is still taught as a kind of 'flopping' and women are urged to let their thoughts wander and day-dream and think about beautiful things, not focusing their minds on anything. This sort of relaxation may not be much use in labour. The auto-suggestion that a woman is required to use to get into this state is so far removed from the reality of the situation – the great muscle of the uterus grinding away like a tremendous dynamo, the stretching of other muscles, the movements of the baby sinking lower, the never-ceasing activity going on within and usually also around her – that, unless she manages to withdraw from her labour entirely and enter into a state of amnesia, labour can be a cruel shock. Even if she succeeds in becoming so amnesic that she does not register pain, she cannot be sensitive to the messages coming from her body. But, in fact, many women who try to drift away from the sensations of labour, and who have never been made aware of the intensity of the feelings they will experience, are unable to escape and are threatened by severe pain once contractions get really powerful. It is only too easy once this has happened to lose confidence, be submerged under waves of contractions, and try to turn and run from your ordeal, or simply to give in and suffer.

Very different from the idea of letting yourself 'flop' is the system of prepared childbirth, which, as we have seen, goes, perhaps unwisely, under the name of *accouchement sans douleur* and 'the psychoprophylactic method', connected with Lamaze, and which was further developed by Pierre Vellay and by Eliza-beth Bing in the USA.

This sort of relaxation, like that taught in the 1930s by Arne Jacobson, is founded on progressive neuro-muscular release, the contraction and release of specific groups of muscles. It is above all *controlled* relaxation, and it demands a woman's alert observation. Although complete, residual relaxation has a place in preparation for the birth, it is complemented by this training in differential relaxation, i.e. the relaxation of groups of muscles, or the contraction of groups of muscles whilst all other muscles not necessary for the movement are relaxed, and by types and rhythms of breathing which can help at different phases of labour.

Psychoprophylaxis included exercises for the limbs which were called 'disassociation'. An exercise of this kind involves, for instance, contracting all the muscles of the right arm, while the rest of the body remains relaxed, or contracting muscles of the right arm and leg, or left arm and leg, while other muscles are 'decontracted'. A woman able to do these exercises well is doubtless very efficient at controlling tension in her body in exercise sessions. (They can be useful to check over your body and limbs to see that they are released when you are finding it difficult to drop off to sleep, for example.) It does not mean, however, that she can relax under stress, and, anyway, she is not required to perform drills of this kind in labour. So such exercises can become something in the nature of conjuring tricks – great fun to do perhaps, but not very useful. In situations of stress we tend to spontaneously contract *muscle groups that act together*, which do not correspond to neat categories such as 'all down the left side' or 'both arms' or 'one arm and the leg on the other side', as in these exercises. Working with muscles in groups which quite naturally act in sympathy with each other is probably more relevant to labour.

Some people think that natural childbirth implies a sort of hypnotic relation between a care-giver and patient and that unless a woman is unusually suggestible this will fail for her. Nothing could be farther from the truth. A woman who is prepared for birth can find this approach works well even if the obstetrician or midwife knows nothing about it at all. But during labour she does need emotional support; a birth companion who understands what she is trying to do should be present and willing to take responsibility, since the mother should not get involved in explanations at this time.

A birth companion's gender may be a secondary consideration. The companion does not, of course, have to be the father of the baby. It is unlikely to be if you are lesbian with a self-inseminated pregnancy. This person must be someone whom you trust absolutely, who understands your priorities, can communicate well, and with whom you can relax and are free to reveal yourself. A tall order!

'Natural childbirth' has meant many different things and has covered every degree of training from the most intensive to the most rudimentary and fragmentary of morale-boosting. It isn't, of course, really natural childbirth. Among human beings all birth is shaped and patterned by culture. It would be better to call this 'prepared' childbirth.

Women sometimes talk about long labours as if they were always ghastly and hope for the shortest labour possible. But long labours can be pleasant and brief labours can sometimes be unpleasant because they are shocking. They also often believe that giving birth to a large baby is bound to be difficult. Yet women can have marvellous experiences giving birth to huge babies or small babies.

Physiological criteria are not the only factors. The important thing about a labour – apart from the one factor which we are in no danger of underestimating, of having a live mother and baby – is how the woman copes with it, and how she emerges from the experience, the effect it has on her mind. This is as much a matter for serious scientific inquiry as are all the physiological criteria which are usually applied. A woman's feelings about the birth are just as relevant. We are dealing here with two orders of reality – the physical facts and the psychological facts. In any birth they are intertwined with, and act and react on, each other.

A leading obstetrician once remarked to me that many women misrepresented their labours. One woman in his hospital was talking about her two previous frightful labours, and the complicated manoeuvres to which the obstetrician had recourse 'to get it away'. From interest he looked up her records, and discovered, he said, that she had had two spontaneous births. He felt that this showed how untruthful women were liable to be. I was more interested in the state of mind of a woman who believed that she had had difficult births. Is it not likely that, however easy these births were from the doctor's point of view, for her they were difficult? However the births appeared to the doctors, for her they were distressing. It seems to me important to accept the validity of a woman's emotional experience.

On the other hand, a woman having an apparently bad labour who seems physically near the end of her tether can yet say, in the middle of that labour, 'It's wonderful.' This is something which we do not fully understand. It has been suggested that it is a form of 'sub-hypnosis', but since this suggests that the woman is in a state of semi-trance, and subject to the influence of another person, the removal of whose presence would result in pain and distress, the term is misleading.

With whatever satisfaction is associated, and whatever name we give it, it is a strange materialism which evaluates birth according to purely physical standards unrelated to the state of mind of the woman who is bearing the child. She is not just a machine through which a baby is brought to birth, a convenient receptacle for the developing fetus in pregnancy, which at the time of labour offers more or less resistance to the child's entry into the world. Her body is part of a *person* for whom the birth of the baby is of major emotional significance. It is the aim of this book to help women experience childbirth with serenity and joy, and gain from it a sense of achievement and deep happiness.

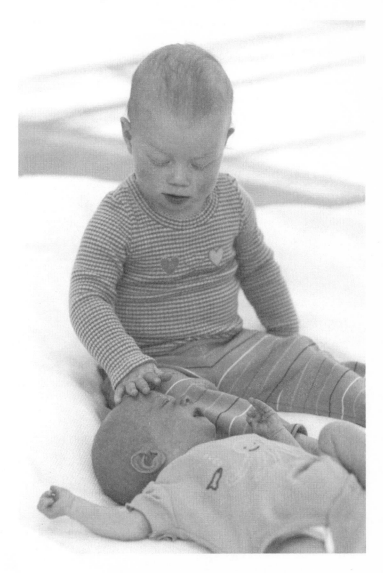

For an older sibling adapting to the baby is an important part of social learning.

3

Pregnancy

FERTILISATION

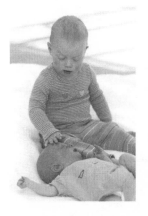

Fertilisation occurs when the sperm buries itself inside the wall of one of the female ova, or eggs, which grow in pockets inside the ovaries. The ova are the largest cells in the human body, but even so they are only 0.2 millimetres in diameter. Each month a ripe ovum is freed from the ovary and starts a journey along the uterine tube towards the uterus. Unless it meets a sperm, it is expelled still unfertilised, but if it becomes fertilised it stays in the uterus and grows into a baby.

Sperms grow inside the testicles and are ejaculated into the woman's vagina in the semen. Each sperm has a flattened, oval head and a long lashing tail, rather like a miniature tadpole, and is between 52 and 62 thousandths of a millimetre long.

Once the ovum is fertilised it starts to segment until it is a mass of tightly packed cells called the morula, like a blackberry. The outer ones are called the trophoblast and form a container for the inner ones which create the embryo.

Liquid is formed between these two sorts of cells. The inside section of the inner cells (the entoderm) now turns into a yolk-sac, and then this entoderm separates from the outer layer (ecto-derm), each drawing aside from the other, and a third layer of germ cells (the mesoderm) is formed between them. The outside layer forms the baby's nervous system, the epidermis of the skin, the sweat glands, oil glands and mammary glands, the hair, nails, nose, mouth, eyes, and some other organs. The inside layer forms the digestive tract and glands, the auditory tubes, lungs, bladder and parts of the thyroid and thymus glands. The middle layer forms the skeleton, muscles, circulatory system and other parts of the body.

By the end of the third week after fertilisation two longitudinal folds have formed in the outside layer, called the neural folds, with the dip between them called the neural groove. The groove has got deeper and the folds have closed over it to make a tube, the neural tube, and where the baby's brain will be there are three bumps, the sites of the forebrain, midbrain and hindbrain. The long part of the tube forms the spinal cord.

Along the front of the neural tube a thick ridge grows (the notochord), from the future midbrain right down to where the vertebral column will later grow.

Part of the yolk-sac is embedded in the embryo at the umbilicus. The embryo is enclosed in a sac of membranes and floats in amniotic fluid which both protects it and allows it to move.

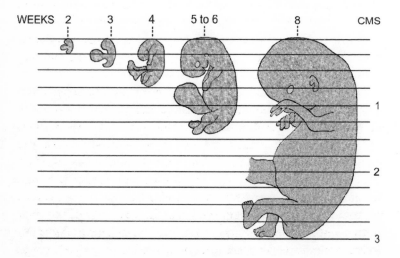

Relative sizes of the embryo from two to eight weeks after conception.

After about a week in the uterine tube the fertilised ovum reaches the uterus and buries itself in the lining. It is this lining which is released every month in the menstrual period. The outside layer of cells of the embryo throws out processes (villi) which dig into the walls of the uterus and get nutrition for the developing embryo from them. At first these villi cover the whole outer layer of cells, but after the end of the second month they atrophy, except at the site of the placenta.

THE FUNCTION OF THE PLACENTA

The placenta is the baby's life support system. The outer layer has short branches, like the stalk structure on a bunch of grapes, which penetrate the maternal tissues. It is through the placenta that the fetus is nourished, oxygenated, and excretes its waste after the first two months of pregnancy. The thin walls of the villi separate the fetal bloodstream from the mother's blood, but the fetus absorbs oxygen and nutrition through them and can excrete its waste material through their delicate walls. Although the baby gets its oxygen and is fed through the mother's bloodstream, there is no direct passage of blood between the mother and the baby or the baby and the mother. The baby is nourished by her through a process of osmosis – that is, some constituents of her blood percolate through to the baby. Many substances which would be harmful to the baby are sieved off in this way so that they never reach it.

The placenta manufactures the sex hormones oestrogen and progesterone, too. Oestrogen causes growth in uterine muscles and the blood vessels in the walls of the uterus that supply them with oxygen. It also causes softening in pelvic ligaments and the vagina and develops milk glands in the breasts.

The placenta usually lies at the top of the uterus. The umbilical cord connects the fetus to the placenta. After the birth of the baby the placenta is expelled and the openings of the torn uterine vessels are shut by contraction of the muscle fibres of the uterine walls; otherwise haemorrhage would result. By this time the placenta is a disc-shaped mass with a diameter of 18-20 cms, and a thickness at the middle of about 3 cms. It looks like a large piece of raw liver. The umbilical cord is attached somewhere near the middle.

YOUR PELVIS

The pelvic girdle is formed by the hip-bones in a shape something like a lobster-pot sloping downwards and forwards, through which the baby passes when being born. The pelvic outlet is limited by the sub-pubic arch in front, the ischial tuberosities at the sides and the sacrum behind. The coccyx, the little bone at the bottom of the spine, although curved forward, is attached to the sacrum by a joint which moves back when the baby is being born, so that it does not get in the way.

Most pelves present no difficulties in childbirth and provide ample room for the baby. Antenatal examination can indicate whether there is likely to be any problem with a malformed pelvis and a large baby. But usually the shape of the pelvis allows a straightforward labour.

The pelvis is not a rigid structure. It is flexible and can spread wide to let the baby through, especially if you squat, kneel or stand, legs well apart, rocking or circling it. So movement is

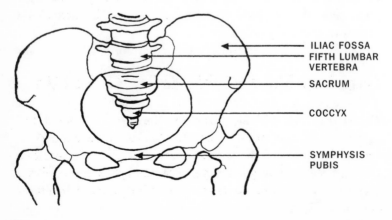

ILIAC FOSSA
FIFTH LUMBAR
VERTEBRA
SACRUM

COCCYX

SYMPHYSIS
PUBIS

The pelvis

vital. If you are stuck in bed labour is more difficult – prolonged and painful – and if you are stranded like a beetle on its back when you are pushing it is harder to get the baby out. Being supine makes it harder for the baby, too, because the oxygen supply is reduced and fetal heart decelerations may result simply because the mother is on her back.

YOUR UTERUS

Your reproductive organs are composed of a hollow, thick-walled muscular uterus, or womb, shaped like a pear with the stalk end pointing downwards and usually slightly backwards. In front and behind are the bladder and the rectum, and the mouth of the uterus, or cervix, connects with the vagina below. From the upper part of the uterus two tubes or oviducts, each about ten centimetres long, run towards the small almond-shaped ovaries which lie on either side.

By the end of pregnancy your uterus has moved up out of the pelvis into the abdomen, is marrow-shaped and about 30 cms long. Its fundus (the top) reaches nearly as high as the dia-phragm, the sheet of muscle which separates the abdomen from the thorax (chest). The baby is protected within the walls of the uterus which are about 1-2 cms thick, and is also inside a bag of membranes, floating in a sea of *liquor*[1] *amnii* (the 'waters'), attached by the umbilical cord to the placenta, through which nourishment flows.

THE DEVELOPMENT OF THE FETUS

Three weeks: The ovum is the size of a small grape. No human characteristics can be recognised.

Four weeks: The sac is 2-3 cms long, about the size of a pigeon's egg. The embryo is curved like a broad bean so that head and tail almost

---

[1] The first syllable rhymes with 'hike'.

meet. The rudimentary eyes are visible and small buds indicate where limbs will develop.

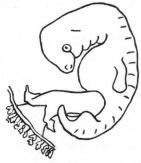

Sketch of the embryo at about a month old. At this stage the developing embryo still looks much like a baby sea-horse. Notice the eye, the rudimentary limbs, nose and mouth.

Eight weeks: The sac is the size of a hen's egg. The placenta begins to grow. Hands and feet are recognisable. The head is large in proportion to the body.

Twelve weeks: The sac is the size of a goose egg and the placenta, which is now well formed, weighs more than the fetus. The fetus weighs about 58 grammes. Fingers and toes are evident.

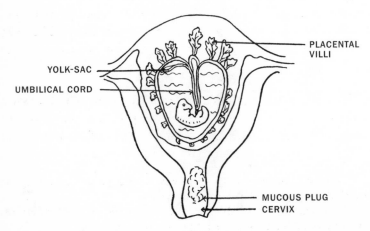

Diagram of the uterus in the first months of pregnancy

Sixteen weeks:	The fetus measures 15 cms and weighs approximately 174 grammes. There is a good heartbeat, but it cannot yet be heard on abdominal auscultation. Fetal movements are present. Sex can be distinguished. Meconium[2] is present in the intestine.
Twenty weeks:	The fetus is about 20 cms long and weighs 290 grammes. *Vernix caseosa*[3] is on the skin and there are fine downy hairs on the head and eyebrows. Fingernails can be distinguished. Fetal movement is felt by the mother (quickening) and the heart can be heard.
Twenty-four weeks:	The fetus measures 30.5 cms and weighs about 464 grammes.
Twenty-eight weeks:	The fetus measures 35.5 cms and weighs 928 grammes.
Thirty-two weeks:	The fetus measures 40.5 cms and weighs 1810 grammes. The skin is red and wrinkled. Lanugo[4] is plentiful.
Thirty-six weeks:	The fetus is 45 cms long and weighs 2720 grammes. There is a little subcutaneous fat. The nails reach the fingertips and the cartilage of the ears is soft.
Forty weeks:	The fetus measures 50 cms or more and weighs 3000 grammes or more. The baby is well covered with subcutaneous fat and the skin is red, but not wrinkled.

You begin to feel your baby moving at any time between sixteen and twenty weeks, usually early with second and subsequent babies, as you already know what it feels like. Some

---

[2] The baby's first stools. They are very dark green and after birth are expelled from the bowel during the first few days.

[3] A substance very much like cold cream or cottage cheese which protects the baby's skin. It may or may not be present at birth.

[4] Fine, downy hairs on the baby's body.

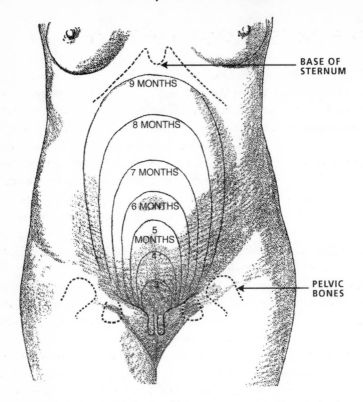

The approximate height of the fundus of the uterus in pregnancy. Notice the descent after engagement.

women say it feels like butterflies; some think it is more like a goldfish swimming round; others feel a soft thudding or something akin to a slight electric shock. It is more noticeable when you relax, especially when you lie down at night and are about to go to sleep.

Be aware of the baby's movements. Your baby probably has a more or less regular energetic kicking time. If you go two or three days without noticing movements, tell your midwife, who will probably suggest that you go to the hospital to check the baby's heart with ultrasound. This is especially important if you go past your estimated date of birth.

THE PHYSIOLOGY OF BIRTH

When labour starts, rhythmically recurring contractions of the uterus gradually dilate the cervix, which is already soft and stretchy as a result of hormone activity. These contractions have been estimated to exert a pressure of about 2 kilos per sq. centimetre. The cervix is pulled open and the lower segment stretched until the completion of the first stage of labour, by which time it has been completely effaced. This is by far the longest stage of labour and, if you are having your first baby, usually takes between about six and thirteen hours, although some women are much quicker and some much slower, and some are not aware of the beginnings of dilatation. In the case of a heavy baby, labour may be a little longer. With subsequent babies labour is usually more rapid. The first stage may last from about four to about eight hours, but there is great variation. The baby's head, flexed forwards on to its chest, is pressed down into the lower segment of the uterus.

When full dilatation occurs the cervix is sufficiently wide open to allow the passage of the presenting part (usually the head). At this point expulsive contractions, with or without the voluntary help of the mother, have the effect of pushing the baby down the birth canal. First the baby's head is pressed down towards her back to get through the pelvic cavity. It is

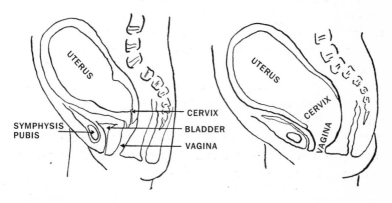

Uterus before labour starts   Uterus when the baby is born

flexed even more and rotates at approximately a right angle. As the head reaches the pelvic floor muscles and the perineum starts to bulge out internal rotation is complete. The head then passes beneath the *symphysis pubis* (the pubic arch). Then the perineum slips back over the face and under the chin and the baby's head turns to come in line with the shoulders, rotating again through an approximate right angle. The shoulder nearest the mother's abdomen is born first, and then the other shoulder. After this the baby's body slips out. The second stage usually lasts from a few minutes to about an hour – or occasionally two hours – and does not usually last longer than about half an hour with a woman having her second or later baby.

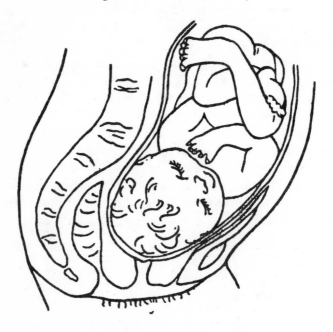

The Baby Before Labour Begins

The baby's head turns towards the mother's back to enter the brim of the pelvis.

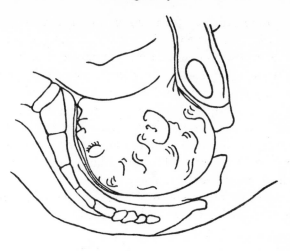

The Birth of the Baby: 1

In the second stage the baby's head is flexed well forward on to its chest as it descends through the birth canal. The head is caused to rotate and the occiput (the back of the head) is in an anterior position, so that the baby is facing the mother's back. As the head reaches the pelvic floor the perineum starts to bulge forward.

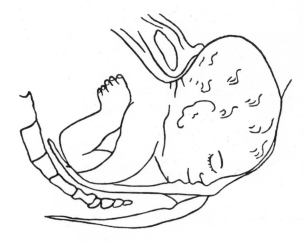

The Birth of the Baby: 2

The birth of the head by extension. The baby's head crowns. Notice that the baby's chin is now lifted well up off its chest.

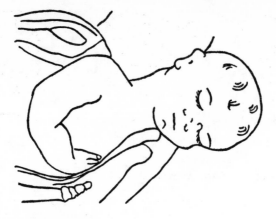

The Birth of the Baby: 3

The baby's head slips out and starts to turn to come into line with the shoulders which are still inside. It passes through approximately a right angle. This is called 'external rotation' or 'restitution'. It all happens quite naturally without assistance. The baby's skin is purplish-blue.

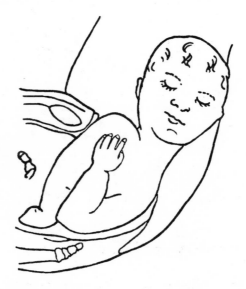

The Birth of the Baby: 4

The anterior shoulder (i.e. the one nearest the mother's abdomen) is born first. Then the rest of the baby's body slides out.

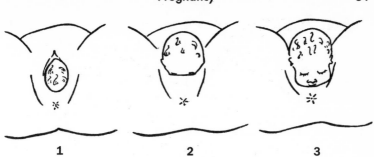

1   2   3

The Birth of the Baby's Head in More Detail

1. The assistants and the partner can see the baby's head at each contraction, but it disappears again between contractions. The perineum is being slowly and gently dilated.
2. The head crowns, and the mother may be able to look down and see it if she is in a suitable position.
3. The head oozes out.

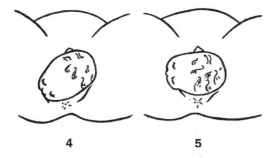

4   5

4. The head begins to rotate externally to come into line with the shoulders which are not yet born. This happens between contractions or at the start of the next contraction.
5. At this point the mother can see her baby's face for the first time.

YOUR PELVIC FLOOR

The sheet of muscles across the floor of the pelvic cavity is called the pelvic floor. The muscles are often used only unconsciously or involuntarily, in defecation and micturition (passing water), and when a woman is mounting to orgasm. Some women are not aware that they possess them. It has been said[5] that 'the term "floor" is not a good one, since it leads one to think of the floor of a house, e.g. a rigid partition running transversely between walls . . . The pelvic floor has no such structure. It is not a rigid partition; nor does it run transversely. It is elastic and movable, varying in its thickness, its nature, and its slope at various parts, while it runs across a very irregularly shaped space – the outlet of the bony pelvis. It is composed of a variety of tissues, differing in their consistence, their strength, and the firmness of their attachment to the bony wall.'

These muscles forming the floor of the pelvis are even more important than the muscles which form the wall of the abdomen. During early pregnancy and later, after the baby is born when a woman wants to get her figure back, she is very conscious of the abdominal wall and reminds herself to hold it in, and so strengthen the muscles which keep her tummy firm.

But there is far less awareness of the muscles of the pelvic floor. Simply because they are not seen they can easily be forgotten. They are important because they form a base to everything inside the abdomen and pelvis, and if they are allowed to get very lax and strained the uterus can slip down out of place, often giving a woman bad backache and making her tired and irritable, and may drop so low that the uterus even protrudes into the vagina. This is the prolapse of middle age, from which younger women can also suffer. It occurs after any excessive straining, either with frantic bearing down during labour, from constant lifting of heavy objects without correct muscle coordination, or as a result of chronic constipation. In the past it was considered the almost inevitable consequence of repeated child-bearing. This can be remedied by exercise of the voluntary muscles, but if it gets very bad the only cure is surgery.

Helen Heardman[6] likened muscle to elastic, which, instead of losing its power to stretch and recoil by continued use, gains in

---

[5] J. Clarence Webster, *Researches in Female Pelvic Anatomy*, Young J. Pentland, 1892.

[6] *Relaxation and Exercise for Natural Childbirth*, Livingstone, 1956. *A Way to Natural Childbirth*, Livingstone, 1948.

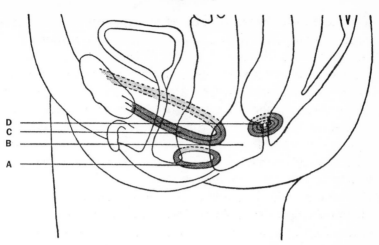

Diagram to illustrate the position of muscles of the pelvic floor over which you can achieve control. The dark shaded ones are those which, with practice, can be felt working.
A. Circular group of muscles round the introitus
B. Crossing network of fibres
C. Muscles which grip and encircle the vagina
D. Muscle which closes the anus

tone as a result of regular exercise. The more muscles are used, the more they can support the internal organs, and the more complete the rehabilitation of the body after childbirth. On the other hand a 'muscle-bound' woman tends to suffer laceration during birth[7] and it is also important that we teach these particular muscles how to 'give'. They form the gateway through which a baby is born into the world, and open up as the head is descending. As the baby slides through the pelvic floor these structures are pulled apart as you might stretch the neck-band of a turtle-neck sweater into which you were wriggling. They do so more easily if you do not offer resistance to the baby's birth. They are already in a more pliable and softer condition, as are many of the tissues of the body, as a result of the action of hormones during pregnancy. In some women these tissues are so soft that they involuntarily pass water when they cough, sneeze

[7] Ballet dancers, keen horse-riders and athletes often find it difficult to release these muscles easily.

or laugh. In this case it is important to practise exercises for the pelvic floor as described in Chapter 5 and to pull in all the muscles of the pelvic floor if you are about to cough.

When you have your postnatal check-up your GP may simply ask, 'Everything all right down below?' If you are in any doubt at all about whether your pelvic floor muscles are well toned, or whether an episiotomy or tear has healed well, ask to be examined. It used to be standard procedure to do a vaginal exam, but this is often neglected now. I think it is rather important, even though nobody wants an unnecessary vaginal examination. It may be that you would benefit from some physiotherapy, and the postnatal check-up is the time to organise this help if you need it.

HOME OR HOSPITAL?

Having a baby does not have to be like a surgical operation, and a woman's attitude of mind is the all-important factor in the ease and spontaneity with which she can give birth. Unless there are reasons why it is best for the baby to be born in hospital, home is usually the best place.

Natural birth is possible in a hospital. But such is the ritual splendour of institutionalised routines in hospital organisation that the woman who hoped to have a natural birth may get bewildered and anxious as staff pop in and out, she is wired up to machines and has drugs pumped into her bloodstream.

Many hospitals fail to offer an environment in which you can focus on the birth, be yourself and do whatever comes spontaneously. The National Childbirth Trust published the results of a Better Birth Environment survey in 2003 based on information from nearly 2000 women in different parts of the UK. Nine out of ten thought the physical surroundings had a big impact on the birth experience and most important was space for moving around, a birth pool or large bath, an en suite toilet, comfortable, adjustable bed (which should not be taking up all the space in the centre of the room), low lights or adjustable lighting, and peace and privacy. More than half said they had no control over who came into the room, and could be overheard by others; there was nowhere pleasant to walk; the room was too clinical; they couldn't get hold of enough pillows, a birth ball or beanbags and floor mats, couldn't control the temperature of the room; and drinks and snacks were not on hand.

Some women, however, are especially afraid of possible complications and of unnecessary pain at home. Psychological reasons for preferring hospital birth must also be taken into account. It may be that as you learn more about childbirth during pregnancy you will come to feel more confident about giving birth at home. You can research home birth by visiting the website www.homebirth.org.uk.

If you want a home birth be prepared for a lot of resistance. Your GP may say that the practice doesn't do them. A doctor's responsibility is to refer you to another doctor who does, in this case. In the UK you have a right to choose where you give birth. Even so, friends, colleagues and relatives may all express misgivings. As one woman said, 'Most people's reaction upon hearing of our home birth was, "Well, I didn't think it was allowed these days" or "My doctor doesn't do home deliveries", or "Dear God, you must be brave staying at home!"' And she added, 'I think the ones going into hospital are the brave ones if the truth were known!'

Having a baby at home need not be costly. The main expense is secondary to the birth itself and is connected with getting adequate help for the 'lying in', as it used to be called. This means nowadays that period of time during which you both concentrate exclusively on the baby and do not bother much with cleaning up or unnecessary cooking. If you plan to spend that time together in a leisurely holiday atmosphere, eating simply prepared food and not trying to follow a clockwork routine, you can thoroughly enjoy yourself. Think of it as a 'baby-moon'.[8] If you have other children already it will have to be a modified kind of baby-moon, with picnics in the bedroom and special treats.

---

[8] Sheila Kitzinger, *Birth Your Way: Choosing Birth at Home or in a Birth Centre*, Dorling Kindersley, 2002.

SOME ADVANTAGES OF HAVING A BABY AT HOME

Perhaps one of the most important reasons for having a home birth is that you are in the security of an environment with which you are familiar and which you control. You are not exposed to the institutional violence that is all too common in some large hospitals in which women are processed through childbirth like products on a conveyor belt, and you are not at risk of becoming an experimental subject for drugs to kick-start and rev up the uterus. The whole process seems more natural and you are far less likely to be traumatised by birth. Labour may appear to be shorter, since you do not commit yourself to it so early, but carry on with normal activities. You have privacy – something which many women value highly – which, unless you are in a private room, you cannot have in hospital, and even in a private room staff may come and go, and you encounter total strangers. At home you are likely to have the concentrated individual care of a midwife whom you already know. An additional, and to many women not inconsiderable, advantage with home birth is that you are not left alone in labour. Someone, either the midwife or your partner, is always with you.

Contrary to general opinion, I think that compared with hospital the mother at home probably has more peace and quiet. She is not troubled by the events and distress of any other woman's labour, as she may be in hospital. She usually gets more opportunity to sleep and relax after the birth, since there is no hospital schedule to be rigidly followed. She is treated as an individual and not expected to conform to a pattern for the ease of running a large and often ill-planned and understaffed ward. She can have her baby with her, cuddle and feed him or her when she likes, and get to know and understand this new little human being. She will not be handed a bottle of made-up artificial baby milk – provided free to the hospital by the manufacturer – just in case she worries that she does not have enough breastmilk. She can see that her baby is not given water – which may satisfy thirst without stimulating the supply of breastmilk by repeated sucking. The baby is not left to cry, and tends to be more peaceful than the hospital baby. The dangers of cross-infection are also avoided. These are very real in many maternity units. She can rest when she wants to without having to fit in with ward routines, move about when she feels like it, and is not propped up in a sitting position in bed, immobility being a contributory factor in thrombosis. Nor if the birth has been difficult is she routinely given painkilling drugs that may pass through her breastmilk to the baby, and which, unless they are carefully monitored, can affect her own nervous system and make her feel confused.

The father, too, has a much bigger share in the first days of the baby's life than if a woman is in hospital. He knows that he is necessary to his partner and child and is not treated as a germ-ridden intruder. And the mother can see her friends and relatives when she likes instead of at set visiting times.

But maybe the upset of a home birth is not really worth it? Some people think that the whole house needs to be re-organised to have a baby at home – but this is far from the truth, and midwives do as little as possible to disrupt the normal running of the home. A hundred years ago things were different, and those who considered they were merely taking adequate precautions against infection used to strip the room where the confinement was to take place of all hangings, curtains and carpets, remove pictures, ornaments and books, and turn it into a sort of operating theatre. My mother was a mid-wife after the First World War and told me that a sulphur candle would be burned in the room in order to sterilise it, and all doors and windows were sealed to keep out germs and dust. When a woman was in labour the seals were broken and she lay on a high bed in the middle of the room with a board placed under the mattress to make it firm, and a roller towel strung round the bed-posts for her to pull and strain on. After the baby was born she had to go on sleeping in her single bed and her husband was not allowed to sleep beside her. Often she had to lie flat for a number of hours or even days after the confinement, and was not permitted to get out of bed for a fortnight. For six weeks after she was still something of an invalid. She was tightly bound up in a binder or large towel wound round her abdomen because it was thought that this would help to get her figure back, but was not permitted to do any exercises.[9]

In an effort to breastfeed the baby she was urged to consume vast quantities of liquid and bottle upon bottle of stout,[10] and often was allowed neither fruit nor vegetables, and certainly not salads, as they were thought to give the baby wind. With lack of any form of muscular exercise and a poor diet she must very often have suffered from constipation, and this was and still is considered by some people a quite normal sequel of childbirth.

Nowadays, at home, when a woman thinks she may be in labour, apart from seeing that everything is ready, she continues with her normal daily routine until she feels that the moment has arrived when she wants to concentrate on her labour. By this time she is probably already half dilated, and the apparent length of her labour has been shortened simply because she has been up and about and her mind has been occupied. She goes to her familiar room surrounded by the furniture, books and pictures she likes. The couple sit or stroll around quietly together, chatting between contractions, and, when they are big enough to need coping with, working together to respond to them smoothly. The midwife, often a friend already, looks in to see that everything is all right and tells them how far the cervix is dilated. They listen to the baby's heartbeat and are very thrilled. The midwife may go away again, leaving her phone number so that they can get her quickly. Some time later they realise that they are approaching the end of the first stage; her partner has made drinks for her and fetched ice from the fridge to refresh and cool her and rung up the midwife to tell her that things are really moving. She arrives, and they form a team working

---

[9] Free movement rather than immobilisation of the abdominal muscles is the quickest way to get your figure back.

[10] Drinking much more than you want is likely to diminish rather than to increase the milk supply. You are naturally thirsty when nursing, but there is no need to drink more than you wish. Water, milk, cocoa, malt drinks, fruit juices, beer, wine – even champagne – are all suitable.

harmoniously towards the same end. There is little need for talk, as each understands what the other is trying to do. The room is very peaceful; there is only the sound of the mother's careful rhythmic breathing and an occasional word of encouragement or advice from her partner or the midwife.

The woman is cold, and her partner brings an extra duvet and a hot water bottle and helps her move to ease the backache as her baby's head presses lower. She loses the rhythm of her breathing a moment and perhaps they breathe together.

At last she feels she must push and, with her partner's arm around her, she starts pressing the baby gently but firmly down the birth canal. Soon the head is visible, perhaps even before she realises that the birth is so near. Her partner may see it first and his eyes are shining with excitement and joy as he tells her. Then she, too, looks down with the next contraction. Before long the whole body slides out. She holds the baby immediately, and the baby is tucked up close to her, while the midwife clears up, and the partner boils the kettle for tea – or opens a bottle of champagne!

The couple are left with their baby, alone in the quiet house, sharing an indescribable sense of wonder. There is an almost honeymoon atmosphere about those first days after the baby has come. The midwife comes in each day to see the baby, take the mother's temperature and blood pressure, examine her sanitary pad in case there are signs of heavy bleeding or infection, and give any advice on feeding the baby that may be needed.

In the familiar surroundings of home the mother is relaxed. She sleeps well, adapts herself to the baby's rhythm rather than to that imposed by hospital routine, and gradually gets to know her child and to plan her day. There is no sudden break, as when a woman comes out of hospital and tries to cope with housework and a baby whom she may not really know up to that time.

PREPARING FOR BIRTH

If you are having a home birth get everything ready three weeks in advance, on a trolley or table, covered by cling-film or a towel. As well as jam-jars (usually for a nail-brush and a thermometer), and bowls which will be on the midwife's list you may like to have:

> T-shirt or short nightdress for labour. Other pyjamas or nightdresses for changing into afterwards.
>
> Bed socks, when the baby is to be born in winter.
>
> An electric heating pad with a plastic cover or a couple of hot water bottles.
>
> An electric kettle in the room or a room nearby.
>
> Raspberry leaf tea[11] and fruit juice.
>
> Barley sugar, glucose tablets or sugar lumps to suck, or honey if preferred.
>
> A small new sponge to soak with iced water for refreshing you at the end of the first stage.
>
> Eau de cologne, cold from the fridge.
>
> Extra towels and a couple of blankets or rugs in cold weather.
>
> An extra lamp that gives good light which can be tilted for the birth so that it does not shine in your eyes.
>
> Three or four extra pillows, or a large floor cushion or beanbag.
>
> A pedal bin for dirty swabs.
>
> Disposal bags for soiled sanitary pads, etc. Disposable nappies. If you have decided to use washable nappies, disposable ones are still useful. They can be torn in half, and put inside a cloth nappy, to prevent excessive soiling.

The bed – preferably a divan without a footboard – should be pulled out from the wall so that there is space on both sides and

---

[11] Raspberry leaf tea has an effect upon the muscles of the uterus. See B. Whitehouse, *Br. Med. J.*, 1,370, 1941; J. H. Burn and E. R. Fell, *J. Pharmacolog.*, 6,785, 1954. It is best taken without milk and with lemon juice if liked, from the seventh month of pregnancy onwards, once or twice daily.

at the foot of it. You may not want to use it at all, but if you do, the mattress needs to be firm, and is best covered with plastic sheeting.

Wherever you plan to have the baby, think ahead to meals after the birth. Ready-cooked dishes can be stacked in the freezer. Plan meals roughly for three days after the birth, and see that ingredients are on hand.

Almond or baby oil is needed for the baby's skin, especially for the buttocks and the cracks which newborn babies often have behind their ears and in the folds of the neck, arms and legs. Talc tends to cake up.

Some nipple cream is useful if you get sore with the first feeds. Best avoid any cream containing peanut oil – arachis oil in the list of ingredients – as this may be associated with a child's later peanut allergy.

Consider hiring a doula, a hired birth companion who will give practical and emotional support in childbirth, and may also offer postnatal support and practical help to you and your family in the first few days or weeks after the birth. One man wrote, 'Having the assistance of Caroline, our doula, meant that I could concentrate all my efforts on supporting my partner, making the birth of our baby girl the most memorable experience of my life. It was a most amazing experience. Having a doula meant I did not need to worry about anything . . . The co-ordination of everything – we did not have to talk too much – it all ran so well.' A woman who hired a postnatal doula wrote, 'It was my doula who helped me say no to the queue of visitors. It was she who helped me stand up to the barrage of opinion from other people and who, with her quiet knowledge, showed me how to be with my baby and take my cues from her.' I used to think that we did not need doulas in the UK, because we have midwives. But at present we cannot rely on having one-to-one care from busy midwives who must try to look after three or even four women at a time, especially in high-tech hospitals where they also have to service and record data from technical equipment. There is powerful evidence that having a woman with you who is not part of the hospital institution, and who focuses on giving you one-to-one continuing support, makes birth more satisfying, and safer for both mother and baby. For the full text and overview of Cochrane Review Continuous Support for Women in Childbirth, 2003, visit www.maternitywise.org/prof/laborsupport. Visit the doula website to find out more: www.doula.org.uk.

Research the childbirth classes you want to attend. The National Childbirth Trust has teachers all over the country. Their approach is eclectic, incorporating the best of different methods of preparation. The website is www.nctpregnancy andbabycare.com. You can locate your nearest classes and send an email to find out about particular courses and check the availability of classes. You can ring 0870 444 8707, too.

Janet Balaskas trained as an NCT teacher and went on to found the Active Birth Movement. The term 'active birth' is a counterbalance to 'active management' by obstetricians. Active birth puts you in charge, not the medical system, but does not rule out medical help when it is needed. A woman gives active birth rather than being a passive patient. She moves around freely and gives birth in an upright or all fours position. Many active birth exercises are based on yoga. To find out where there are classes ring 020 7281 6760 or visit www.activebirth centre.com

Consider having a water birth. This could be in a hospital where there are pools. Find a hospital with more than one pool if possible – where there is only one pool, it is often being used when you want it. Or you could hire a pool to install at home. For information about hiring a pool email mail@active birthcentre.demon.co.uk or ring 020 7281 6760.

One woman told me, 'As soon as I got into the water I felt safe, secure, free. The water cradled me. I wasn't heavy any longer – and I could move.' Research shows that women who are immersed in water during the first stage of labour are significantly less likely to want drugs for pain relief. So even if you do not plan to give birth in water, being in a pool, with the water over your tummy, may make labour much less painful. Midwives who assist at water births develop an understanding of birth that is denied those who work in hospitals where it is the practice to hurry birth and tell women when and how to push.

As one midwife said, 'Water births are peaceful. There's no need for commanded pushing. The mothers seem much more confident that what they are doing is right.' Another told me, 'The perineum is usually protected by the water. As a result an episiotomy (cutting the perineum to enlarge the birth opening) is rarely needed.' No randomised controlled trials have demonstrated that this is the case, but it is likely that when a woman is in a pool it affects practice, and a midwife is less quick to intervene.

The Council that regulates midwives in the UK has made it clear that every midwife should be able to care for women having water births. It is not an unusual skill that only some midwives have. So you should not be prevented from being in water because the hospital does not have a specially trained midwife available. In practice, however, many midwives are anxious about water births and try to avoid them. They may say that someone else is using the pool when they are not, that the pool has not been cleaned yet, that it will take too long to fill it (twenty minutes), or produce medical reasons why you cannot use it. Having raised blood pressure should not be one of these. Immersion in warm water lowers blood pressure, though there may be a hospital rule that women with hypertension cannot be in the pool. But one valid reason for not having a water birth is if you have had an injection of opiates – these drugs may cause respiratory depression in the baby.

THE DISPLACED SIBLING

If there are already children in the family, the introduction of the new brother or sister is made much more easily at home. During labour older children can go in and out of the room or, if they want to be with you and to see the birth, they can stay, though each child should have an adult who takes personal responsibility, so that you can concentrate on what you are doing. They can touch the new baby and help with its bath. This is much more fun than playing with dolls! Birth is accepted more naturally by the siblings, and is not thought of as an illness for which you have to rush to hospital. Since many babies are born at night, a toddler may be tucked up in bed before you start your labour in earnest. Or you may feel most relaxed if you have your other children around, and consider it an important experience for them, and a natural part of your life as a family. This not only affects the acceptance of the new baby by an older child, but the continuing loving relationship between you, which is not suddenly threatened by your withdrawal at a moment of family crisis, the excitement of which a small child must sense.

When the older child meets the new baby you can point out the tiny nails and eyelashes and talk about how little and helpless the baby is. Allow the first expressions of joy in the baby's birth to come from the child. If a doll or some other special present is waiting to celebrate the birthday the advent of the baby is made even more welcome. A toddler can be cuddled at the same time as the baby, and if a special store of biscuits or fruit is kept for feeding times, and toys and other materials for quiet occupations are in your room, they can be very pleasant and looked forward to, rather than being resented by the displaced child. Take time to give positive encouragement and help to hold the baby correctly. By no word or action should you suggest that the older child intends to hurt the baby.

When grandparents, relations and other visitors arrive, a toddler who enjoys it can be the person who takes them to the new baby. In this way the baby belongs to the older child too, and is not simply a rival.

All these things are difficult or impossible to organise in hospital, and the resulting jealousy is likely to be more acute and painful for the toddler and difficult for you to cope with in the early weeks, when you least want to be troubled with psychological problems of this kind, and have little time to deal with them.

But however well parents have organised the birth and care of the toddler, and however careful to give plenty of attention and make him feel loved and wanted, do not feel that you have a maladjusted child, or that you are hopeless failures as parents, if the toddler shows overt or concealed jealousy later, perhaps when the baby is beginning to acquire new skills and is the object of much adult attention as he or she takes the very first steps or says her first words. Some parents feel that in having done all they could to counteract jealousy it should not make its appearance at all, and some forget that it is not only in the early weeks that jealousy may be most apparent, but that it may become noticeable after the baby's novelty has worn off. Sibling jealousy is a natural phenomenon and one that parents must expect to confront. Whilst removing the baby from danger, it is important to face up to any shock or horror you may feel at signs of jealousy. Shock is an unhelpful emotion and inhibits positive action. Home birth does not eliminate sibling jealousy, but it can defer its appearance and possibly also lessen its intensity.

Being present at the birth of a sibling can be an important educational experience for a child, one that most children don't get an opportunity to have. Most of them learn about birth only by watching TV or in 'sex ed' lessons at school. One mother told me about her three-year-old's role in her labour, 'He rubbed my back during contractions. After Molly was born he knelt down beside me and hugged me and said, "You got the baby out very well, Mummy."' Another woman described her two-year-old's enthusiastic participation, 'When Daisy came out he was yelling "Bubby! Bubby!" He then helped cut the cord. Having him there helped me as his presence kept me calm and more controlled. He was more than observer, as he helped by spraying me with water. He felt part of it. I wasn't sure how much of it he would remember, yet (eight months later) he still speaks about it. I feel that having him there helped him accept his sister. He knew where she came from. I haven't had the usual jealousy problems and he is very protective of Daisy.' Anna is thirteen and wrote to me about her experience of the birth of her sister when she was six years old. 'Her birth is one of my most vivid and exciting memories and I realise now that I was lucky being able to share that special day with my Mum and Dad and, of course, Rachel.'

To conclude: The birth of a child is a *family* event and when it takes place at home is a normal part of life. If you are looking ahead to what you hope will be a normal birth, home may be the best place.

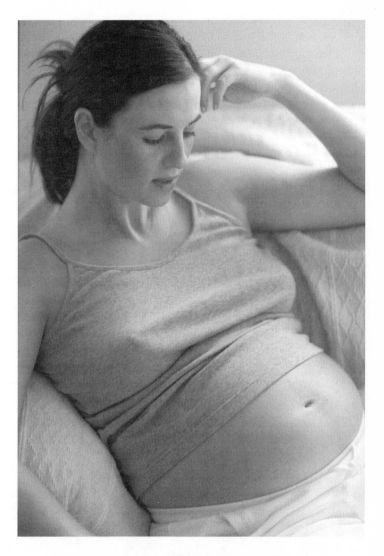

Bringing new life into the world stimulates hope and awe at the unfolding miracle but brings fears and doubts too.

4

The Psychology of Pregnancy

EMOTIONS IN PREGNANCY

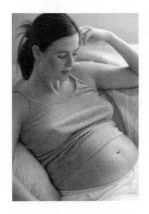

Here we are concerned not with the physical development of the fetus and the birth of the baby, but with feelings about having a baby which any of us may have.

We hear a great deal about the increased sensitivity of the pregnant woman. By tradition she is unstable, unpredictable, easily driven to tears, with strange, illogical desires and fancies. She is stereotyped as the essence of irrational femininity.

Is it true that she is more emotional? Well, yes and no!

A woman who is preparing herself for childbirth is less likely to suffer from the extremes of emotional unpredictability than one who faces birth ignorant and fearful. But, however knowledgeable a woman and however great her trust in herself, she may be more vulnerable than usual – more quickly disgusted and nauseated by the ugly and the cruel, more readily thrilled by beauty and tenderness. As Christmas comes, to give but one instance, the image of the Child in the manger is for her not the sentimental symbol which it may have been up till then, but brings with it the wonder of the promise of new life and the assurance that 'each child comes into the world with the message that God has not yet despaired of men'.

Difficulty in Adjusting to Pregnancy

However much they dreamed of having a baby, the realisation that they are pregnant comes to many women – especially when the child is conceived within a few months after the start of a relationship and a couple are still taking the first steps in learning to live together – as a shock, and often as one not wholly pleasant. Suddenly you are somebody different – an expectant mother – a subject of interest and concern to society; your life seems to be no longer intimate, but something anybody can talk about. They even know when your last period was and whether you are vomiting in the morning. You go to the antenatal clinic where your urine and blood are tested, blood pressure taken, and you are sounded with stethoscopes and patted and tapped. This is all, to say the least, a sudden, if necessary, invasion of privacy.

A pregnant woman is no longer a girl, like the others in the office; something has set her apart from them now. Remarks are made about her 'condition'. It is not just professional care-givers who intrude on the pregnancy and want to pat and stroke her bump. It seems that anybody and everybody feels they can. As one woman put it: 'I am interested to know why it is women feel the need/right to come up to me and comment on my size. I have a large well-defined bump for my body, but I wonder why women (mostly strangers) keep telling me how huge I look, telling me I look fit to burst etc. No one tells me how great I look, just indirect criticisms. I now also get comments on the fact that I'm over 40 weeks – "Not had that baby yet?" – like I'm failing in some way. I'm sure I'm a little more sensitive and vulnerable at the moment, but I find other people's comments rather upsetting. There seems to be so much competition from women, rather than support.' Perhaps it is a way of trying to share in a pregnancy – somehow getting the magic from a woman who has life developing in her, as in the Middle Ages when people would touch kings to catch their glamour and power. Many women who are unprepared for this transition find themselves confronted with the role of the expectant mother which they are unable or unwilling to play. They are forced to act a part they do not know, one that is sometimes quite frightening.

A woman's main concern may be not to lose her figure too soon and get it back again immediately after the birth. She sees photographs of pop stars and models emerging from the clinic, in which they have just given birth by Caesarean section, looking svelte and sexy – the same media icons who went through pregnancy radiating glamour.

Any difficulty in adjusting to the role of pregnancy is often made harder by the pressures put on her. According to the magazines, she should aim to turn herself into a kaleidoscope of personalities. She should be a career success, bake bread, do a little oil painting in her spare time. She cannot open a magazine without reading how she should make herself over, throw a party, restyle her home, and look stunning at 8 p.m. after having been in the office all day in the same clothes. Now on top of all that she's supposed to juggle kids and a career and turn herself into a super-mum.

When she gets pregnant, society is concerned about her – but not for herself and her achievements – only because she has a baby inside her. She does not matter. The baby does. She is warned to look after herself, not smoke or drink, to rest and eat nourishing food, and she resents feeling merely a vessel for the baby. Sometimes she longs to do something shocking – to ski, or have an affair.

When couples have been together only a short time and did not expect to start a baby so soon, inter-personal problems which could have been slowly worked out over the months may come to a head. If the woman is suffering from severe pregnancy nausea, has varicose veins or haemorrhoids, and her breasts are swollen and aching, and feels that all her physical attractions are being swept away by unwelcome maternity, sex can no longer be the ritual by which quarrels are patched up and through which physical closeness takes the place of understanding between two people who may be finding it hard to adjust to each other. Some women force themselves to have sex, but are unable to experience orgasm.

She may feel that her man will lose interest in her with a body spreading in all directions like this. Unless her partner shares with preparations for the birth and gets interested in the details of the unknown experience that lies before them, she may feel very alone and unwanted. In the words of one pregnant woman, 'We are not going along the same path any longer', or, as another said, 'I'm growing farther and farther away from him'.

Some women suffer the strain of never being able to talk about their pregnancy, the birth, or the new baby, because the man seems to close his mind to it all, ignores the fact that she is pregnant, as far as possible, and tries to act as if it were nothing to do with him anyway and it is all 'a woman's affair'. To such women pregnancy, in spite of wanting the baby, can be an unhappy time.

For other women it is much worse. They feel physically nauseated by the body of the child developing in them like a parasite. They are horrified by the inevitability of the process once it has started, at the thickening of their bodies and the movements of the kicking baby.

It is not only the woman who is obviously distressed who may need help. A woman may be doing fine and taking pregnancy in her stride – asserting, as she downs her third whisky or smokes the twentieth cigarette, that 'it doesn't make any difference to me'. She may confront labour with an over-brisk cheerfulness: 'It's just like shelling peas', or refuse any antenatal preparation and react violently against a concentration of ideas on motherhood and the coming baby with, 'I'm sick and tired of all the talk', or 'Hens don't make all that fuss' (some do).

Straightforward fear of childbirth is not the commonly confronted obstacle that once it was; and, where it persists, accurate information may be all that is required to dispel it. After all, it is safer nowadays to have a baby than to drive in Bank Holiday traffic. But fear often comes disguised under a cloak of apparent nonchalance and sometimes is symptomatic of a deeper anxiety, where the woman feels humiliated or trapped by her pregnancy, or confronts problems which make her liable to depression during, or after, the pregnancy. Unless it is plain that she is severely disturbed, it still happens too often that everyone tries to jolly her out of it: 'It's just hormones', they say and, to her partner: 'Take her to a movie' – which is about as much use as the often recommended glass of wine at bedtime for the non-orgasmic woman.

Whether or not a woman wants the baby, whether she enjoys being pregnant or hates it, her relationship with the professionals who care for her must affect the way she approaches the birth.

A pregnant woman is alert to any suggestion that things may not be quite as they should be. She stores each word uttered by the health professional and goes home to worry about their exact significance. 'We ought to keep an eye on you . . .' Why? Something must be wrong! 'We must check your blood pressure . . .' Am I developing pre-eclampsia . . . ?

You need to be familiar with common medical terms simply to know what doctors and midwives are talking about, since it can be distressing to hear a conversation about your inside in technical terms which you cannot understand. Every woman has a right to know what her care-givers are talking about in front of her and to have any difficulties explained. Medical language creates a screen between them which makes her feel that they have something they want to hide from her.

It is important also for the obstetrician or midwife to take the extra time needed to tell her that her baby is fine and that everything is going splendidly. This gives her an emotional boost instead of the depression she so often feels after a clinic visit. Midwives usually explain things and try to find out what you want to know. But it isn't the same with all obstetricians.

Doctors need to be aware of the impression they have on their patients. Some would be appalled if they realised what they thought about them. I know an obstetrician who prides himself on his sympathy but is described by women as 'unapproachable' and 'always so rushed'.

This is partly due to sheer lack of time. He – and more often than not it is a man – cannot be bothered with inessentials and the niceties of polite conversation when so much that is urgent is waiting to be done. But it is partly due also to the social distance that exists between doctor and patient which maintains his status *vis-à-vis* the lay person and makes his pronouncements worthy of respect. The 'bedside manner' disappeared with the doctor who acted the part of kindly father confessor and avuncular adviser – a role which served to maintain this distance by its assumption of implicit authority and superior status. In his place has come the clinician, the foreman and manager of the baby factory who treats the women lying on the examination tables as if they were so many fish on a slab. The only way in which this can be altered is for women to protest.

Unless and until doctors have the time and skill to interest themselves in the psychological care of pregnant women there will remain a vast field of therapy which is at the moment largely left to chance. David Stafford-Clark in *Psychiatry Today*[1] claimed that if 'the actual proportion of time in the medical curriculum devoted to the teaching of psychiatry . . . were to approach in proportion the size of the problem which the qualified doctor must meet in his practice, a great deal of the existing balance and emphasis in medical training and in medical examinations would have to be changed'.

Midwives, who might find it easier to get closer to women and understand what was going on in their minds, are also hampered by lack of training in psychology except of a rudimentary kind, and by being sucked into a medicalised system of care. But ultimately it is not psychotherapy that we need, but simple human understanding and emotional support.

What about my Job?

In the UK, a woman who is employed, who earns at least £77 (on average) a week, and has notified her employer of the pregnancy by the fifteenth week before the baby is due, cannot be given the sack because she is pregnant, whether she is working full- or part-time. If your work is not suitable for pregnancy you

---

[1] Pelican, 1951.

must be offered alternative work if it is available, for which your pay must not be less. It is illegal to sack you or make you redundant for any maternity-related reason. For information about maternity rights visit the Maternity Alliance website: www.maternityalliance.org.uk. You can also call 0207 490 7638 for advice.

It is very difficult coming to a decision about work when you do not know how you are going to feel after the baby comes, and even whether you will be able to tolerate leaving the baby to be cared for by someone else. It is probably best to leave arrangements flexible and not to decide definitely that you will not return to your job until you see how things turn out. Sometimes certain kinds of work can be organised in your own home, but this needs self-discipline and great energy, the ability to work in the very early morning after the first feed of the day being an undeniable advantage.

A woman who is committed to her career and intends to continue in it following the baby's birth will find that she has to run an obstacle course. Friends and family may assume that she will be a full-time mother, and both men and other women may be critical of her if she is not prepared to devote her time to her baby. Men see her as ambitious and aggressively competing with them, and other women see her as unfairly getting the best of both worlds. I believe that each mother should work out for herself the lifestyle which seems right for her, and the answers cannot be exactly the same for different people. A frustrated, angry woman is unlikely to be a loving mother able to enjoy her baby. If she can, the woman whose career matters to her a great deal should get together with other women in a similar situation to talk things through, and perhaps seek joint solutions. This may be possible through a women's group or just by advertising in a paper for other women in the same situation.

The most important ingredients of a happy mother–baby relationship for a woman who is anxious about getting bogged down in motherhood are flexibility of arrangements and physical mobility. So plan to circumvent the strict timetable for work. For some women there is a chance of freelance or part-time work for the first few years, and they can thus keep a foothold on their careers without having to sacrifice the mothering experience. But even if this is not a practical solution for you, it is worth seeing if you can get work at home whenever possible rather than having to go to an office. If you are working with subordinates, or have a secretary, find out if it is possible for them to come to you at home rather than you fitting into the organisational framework in which you operated before the baby arrived. Do as much as you can on the telephone if you can afford it; arrange for help with the house, cleaning, laundry, shopping and cooking, so that you can spend more time with the baby; rationalise housework and see where machines would help save time and energy; work out with your partner how he can have time with the baby, too, and do his full share of basic chores. Physical mobility means having some control over your own transport, so that you are not dependent on other people's timetables, and having equipment which allows you to take the baby with you whenever practicable. Try not to be embarrassed about asking people for help and not to feel personally rejected if they turn you down. Our society is not organised for mothers and babies, and everything you do is also pioneering for other women.

In the first three years of your baby's life especially, a loving one-to-one relationship is important for his or her emotional development. This does not mean that the mother is the only person who can fill this role, although there is a biological urge for a parent to be spontaneously most deeply involved in the child's welfare. A succession of people who come and go, or large groups of which the small child is just another member, however physically well cared for, are disturbing for the child and inhibit the ability to form close, loving relationships as an adult. So until a child is ready for this arrangement – and only you can judge – a crèche may be less satisfactory than a single mother-substitute. Some couples find that a good solution is for each to be part-time parent and part-time worker outside the home, dove-tailing their jobs so that there are shared responsibilities and opportunities. This is a new pattern of living that may find a much greater place in the future.

When you are making arrangements for care, remember that

after the baby comes you may discover that you are anxious about other people looking after your child for long periods of time, however carefully you had planned it all beforehand. So be prepared for emotional changes in yourself as well.

Depression a Month before the Birth

Towards the end of pregnancy many women suffer unaccountable depression which passes off as suddenly as it came and for no apparent reason. I have noticed that among women attending my classes there is a time between the sixth and the third week before the expected date of birth when fear may flood in; you may find this is the time you are most impatient with pregnancy. This 'stage fright' is normal. Extravagant as it may be, why not buy a new maternity top or earrings when this time comes, to help lift morale? Get out and enjoy some entertainment and recreation. While rest is necessary, try to arrange something to look forward to each day so that your thoughts cease to centre only on your pregnancy and the weight inside you. In my experience this depression prior to the birth is much more common than the 'baby blues'.

By this time you feel weary and long for the baby to come, even if you sailed through the early months. If you have always been active, it can be very irritating to feel impeded and weighed down by your body.

In the last six weeks of pregnancy you may need to adjust to new, slower rhythms. Allow yourself to rest more (if other people will let you) and get 'in tune' with your body. If you cannot do this you risk producing the stress that is associated with raised blood pressure.

Wanting to Kick over the Traces

Any woman who does not make a fetish of training herself for childbirth is bound to want to rebel occasionally, to feel free and undisciplined, forget she is pregnant, eat and drink what she likes, give the exercises a miss.

This is fine. To allow for an occasional week or so when

preparation is neglected, therefore, it is important to begin regular relaxation and breathing as early in pregnancy as possible, any time after the third month. You can then proceed in a leisurely fashion, not being driven on by lack of time before labour takes you unawares.

Thinking about the Baby Inside

The boundaries between a woman and the baby inside her are blurred and shifting. The baby is part of you, yet not you. At first it seems odd, exciting but at the same time eerie, to feel inner movements that you cannot control. It is distressing for some women who dislike being pregnant – like an invasion from outer space. They may picture the baby as a parasite clinging to them or as an enemy within. Right through pregnancy you may veer between feeling the baby as part of yourself, an intimate companion deep inside, and as an intruder. At birth you encounter the astonishing otherness of this little creature, and then, when the child comes to the breast and latches on, the baby becomes again as if part of yourself.

Worries about Disability

A pregnant woman may worry about the baby having a disability. Some women keep the pregnancy a secret from friends, and even family, until after the anomaly scan has revealed that there are no obvious disabilities. They are unable to start bonding with the unborn baby till they are already nearly halfway through pregnancy. Lying awake in the dark, they think, 'What if this thing I am nourishing and cherishing within my own body, around which my whole life is built now, whose heart beats fast deep inside me – what if this child should turn out to be something I should be able to love, but which I will shudder to see?'

It is useless to try to force yourself not to brood on such matters, because the more you push them out of your conscious mind, the more tightly they pack the world of dreams. Every unwise remark made by midwife or doctor seems to confirm your misgivings. 'We ought to keep an eye on you . . .' 'The baby's very small . . .' 'Does it move much . . . ?' Statistics do not reduce your fear. If 997 babies are normal, how much worse it seems for your baby to be abnormal.

This is not a private, individual fear. It is shared by many pregnant women, although a few may laugh at it. Once you realise that you are not alone in this experience you escape from the isolated pain it involves. You are no longer enclosed in yourself, fighting it in darkness.

As their baby slips out into the world, the first question of many new mothers who have experienced this fear is, 'Is it all right?' At this moment they are unmasked. Their question is urgent, imperative. They are not yet aware of the baby as a person – but only as their own offering, squirming out of the darkness. They must see the baby immediately to know for themselves the truth, hold it and see its perfection and whole-ness. No wonder they laugh and cry at the same time.

But new babies do not always look perfect. Sugar-loaf moulding of a persistent occipito-posterior (i.e. the peculiar shape of head and bruising of a baby who has been presenting by the face) – pressure marks, marks of the forceps, haematoma – these are all easily explained by the doctor or midwife, but when a mother does not see her baby straight away she imagines much worse things. She may be so sure that something is wrong that reassurance comes with great difficulty, even when the child is peacefully sucking in her arms and is to all intents and purposes a normal, healthy baby.

Perhaps every pregnant woman has also wondered at some time, maybe in the dead of night when she is most alone, how she would react to her baby being born dead and whether she could face it. For some women it is a nagging fear which holds threat of punishment for negative feelings that they have had about the baby and becoming a mother. Perhaps the baby was conceived before it was really convenient, and the woman thought of having a termination and now feels guilty that she even considered it. Perhaps she was pregnant before, and that pregnancy was terminated, maybe for good reasons, but the abortion casts its shadow forward on to the present pregnancy.

There must be few women who have not thought occasionally that pregnancy was a nuisance or been apprehensive at the thought of having to cope with a baby and the drastic change in lifestyle necessitated by its arrival. Women punish themselves for feelings of rejection with fantasies of the child being born dead or being physically or mentally handicapped. This may be because we have unrealistic ideas about 'maternal instincts'. We anticipate having only loving, happy thoughts of babies and motherhood, but in fact feel just as many conflicting emotions about pregnancy and the baby as about any other challenging life experience that produces stress and which forces us, in spite of ourselves, into new patterns of behaviour and thinking.

It is partly that older people – mothers and mothers-in-law especially – anticipate that a baby will come and 'make' a marriage and that the young couple will 'settle down'. 'June's having a baby' the future grandmother says proudly, as if 'everything is all right now!' . . . 'She's becoming just like me, and I understand all her feelings and everything she's going through, because we're women.' And sometimes the pregnant woman wants to scream, 'It's not like that a bit! I want this child, yes, but not if it means that Jo and I aren't able to feel the same about each other any more. And I don't intend to let it change our lives. And I never, never, mean to become a replica of you!' In having dreadful thoughts that it may be dead, the expectant mother is then resisting her mother's view of her and taking the baby away from the grandmother. Her fear that the baby might be born dead or with a disability may be a side-effect of a turbulent relationship with the older woman.

When it's been Difficult to Conceive

There are special problems for the IVF mother or any woman who has for a long time been trying to conceive or hold on to a pregnancy. She has attended fertility clinics and been through the mill of all the tests, examinations and treatments. Sex has become a means of trying to conceive a child rather than something enjoyable in itself. There have probably been times when she has pleaded with her partner to have sex *now* because her temperature chart has indicated that this is the time of ovulation, but he is tired and feels he is being used like a stud bull.

Once she gets pregnant she may have little confidence in her ability to bear this child and is beset with fears that the baby will be abnormal or that she will lose it during the pregnancy. She may have become highly dependent on hospital staff, too, feeling that if she needed help with conceiving it, how much more likely is she to need obstetric intervention with actually giving birth to the baby. Women who are going through this kind of stress may benefit from belonging to a discussion group where they have the opportunity to talk to and share experiences with other pregnant women. Breathing and relaxation classes are not enough.

ULTRASOUND

When I wrote the earliest editions of this book, obstetric ultrasound had not been invented. Since then ultrasound scans have come to be used routinely in most pregnancies. You can expect at least two scans, one early on to decide when the baby is due and another 'anomaly' scan – to detect whether the baby has any abnormalities – at about twenty weeks while it is still legally possible to have a termination. You may be offered other scans as well to investigate if it is developing normally. This is the same technology as that used by fishing fleets to detect shoals of fish. High–pitched sound waves are bounced off anything solid, which shows up as a picture.

Though it is assumed that you will have whatever is on offer, think about the implications of this technology and decide if it is what you want. With ultrasound the mother's body becomes as if transparent. The modern technology of obstetrics peels away layers of muscle that screen the baby from view to examine the unborn patient. It brings benefits, but with psychological risks, too. I know women who have lived through the rest of the pregnancy anxious about a deviation from the normal that has been picked up by the scan – a cyst in the kidneys, for example, or suggested intra-uterine growth retardation – when the baby has turned out to be perfect and of a good weight. Some women have continued to worry even after the baby's birth.

Be aware that ultrasound results are often tentative and that they depend on whoever is interpreting the images. The probe passes over heart, lungs, kidneys, skull, and the back of the neck to estimate if there is an enlarged sac that introduces a suspicion of Down's syndrome. Exact dimensions are measured. Shadows are explored. Arches and promontories of bone are examined to check whether they have fused. Does the fetus react by movement in response to the shrill whistle of ultrasound that only it can hear?

Many women are certain that they could not cope with an imperfect baby and would want an abortion if anything suspect was disclosed. They may lie awake in the night imagining a child with horrific handicaps. Whatever investigations they are required to go through, they need to *know*. Others are less sure, and may regard serial ultrasound testing (repeated scans) as an ordeal to which they are unwilling to subject themselves. *You* can decide what is right for you.

JEALOUSY

Living, as he did, within a patriarchal society, Freud described a culture in which women envied men for all that they possessed, the symbol of much of this jealousy being crystallised in penis envy. But men envied women not at all, since they were inferior beings anyway. Ian Suttie[2] suggested, however, that men might envy women their power of bearing children, and believed that the practice of 'couvade' (French for hatching) in many indigenous societies of South America and Africa, for example – where the husband is treated as if he and not his wife were having the baby, and goes into labour instead of her – was 'an expression of unconscious desire on the part of the husband to share in the production of the child'. According to

[2] *Origins of Love and Hate*, Kegan Paul, 1935.

the theory, it is jealousy not of the baby, but of the woman's ability to be with child. Suttie calls it 'Zeus jealousy', since Zeus swallowed his pregnant wife in order to bear her child himself.

As the woman becomes more engrossed with her pregnancy, with the fascinating movements of the baby and her dreams of what the child will be like, the man may feel more and more shut out. Unaware of her partner's isolation, she interprets his questions and concern, by which he expresses his desire to enter into her world, as fussiness, and may scorn his care and over-protectiveness. Or he may withdraw into a man's world, as-serting his masculine role aggressively, and take no interest in the pregnancy or in her hopes or fears about the birth.

Couples who prepare together for birth and share the experi-ence are far less likely to have this feeling of separation from each other. He feels that he has helped to make this baby, not only because he scattered sperm and started the growth of the fetus in a split moment of time, but that he is in a much deeper and wider sense the child's creator.

SEX IN PREGNANCY

'Should we make love or not?' . . . 'I'm not enjoying it any more. Will it always be like this?' . . . 'He says I can't love him or I'd want sex when he wants it.' . . . 'The doctor says no sex in case we lose this one. He doesn't know Bill! Already we're getting on each other's nerves and we have another five months of it.' . . . 'He's been put off sex by my pregnancy. Last night I tried to get him to make love. He began to get excited and came inside, and the baby moved, and he said, "Oh! it's alive in there!" And after that he just couldn't.'

Many books on sex neglect the very important subject of sex in pregnancy and after the baby comes, and the developing relationship between a couple as together they create a child.

Intercourse is by no means the whole of a woman's sexual-ity. It is only one aspect, and menstruation, pregnancy, birth and breastfeeding are all part of the totality. There is, for in-stance, an ebb and flow in a woman's sexual desire which closely corresponds to these other functions. They are not isolated each from the other, but interdependent parts of her sexual cycle.

Intercourse can continue throughout pregnancy, with the emphasis on a careful tenderness. Great unhappiness is caused to some women when their men refuse to make love. Some men hate pregnancy because they believe that sex is dangerous. One woman spoke to me of the distress she felt at her partner's refusal to make love because he had read that during the first three months of pregnancy, the last three months and the three months after it, a couple should not have intercourse. He thought that if he allowed himself to penetrate her 'the bag of waters would burst' and premature labour immediately result.

A woman came to me distressed because she had lost her baby at about twelve weeks. She remembered that they had made love just before it happened and asked her GP if that could have been the cause. He casually nodded his head and said, 'Yes. I expect that did it. I expect he bonked the little fellow on the nose!' Not only could this not happen – the fetus is well protected inside the bag of waters – but if, as in this particular case, the woman is tense and anxious anyway, she *may* be more likely to hold on to her pregnancy if she can enjoy lovemaking and relax in her partner's arms.

Usually the penis is not long enough to touch the uterus during intercourse, because as the woman becomes sexually aroused not only do the accordion-like folds in the vagina open up, but the vagina also becomes longer. When she is very excited it becomes tent-shaped.

Women starting childbirth classes often wonder if they will be able to relax in labour and think there must be a special sort of neuro-muscular control – different from anything else they experience – which they have to achieve in labour. In fact, if you are really relaxed in childbirth it is very much like the complete release from tension and the luxurious warmth and peace after happily making love. The expression on a woman's face after a satisfying orgasm is similar to that on the face of one who is enjoying her labour – glowing skin, flushed cheeks and shining eyes, damp and untidy hair, and deep content. Coitus and childbirth create their own sanctuaries from the anxieties and concerns of the surrounding world.

Because it is easy to feel guilty, it is important that each woman should be free to follow her feelings, and not be forced into a pattern of behaviour just because the books or an expert say so. If you have previously miscarried you may want to avoid penetration when the second and third periods are due, for this is the time when you are most likely to miscarry again. Only if there is bleeding during the present pregnancy need penetration be avoided till after the third period has been missed.

As you get larger you can invent new positions so that you are comfortable, and at no time should your partner's whole weight rest on you, or great pressure be put upon the uterus, either from outside or from the conventional position in which he lies at full length on top of you. This is a very poor one for pregnancy, and also for afterwards, when your breasts may be full and tender.

In the first three months of pregnancy the woman has to make terrific emotional and physiological adjustments. The pregnancy affects every cell in her body, and she is becoming a different sort of person in terms of her physical self (she may be very tired, suffering from nausea or bouts of vomiting) and in terms of her feelings about herself and her body.

Some women dislike sex right through pregnancy. But to many the upsurge of happiness that comes with the realisation of pregnancy brings with it intense delight in sex – if not immediately, at least after the difficult first few months when any nausea is over.

It is often assumed that penetration is an essential part of sex for a heterosexual couple. Even so, some women never enjoy penetration as much as clitoral stimulation. Others, who usually welcome it, dislike it towards the end of pregnancy, and fear that it may harm the baby. Furthermore, after the baby has dropped into the pelvis it feels as if there is very little space left. If you think how painful a full bladder can be in the last weeks, you will realise that the erect penis can also cause pain unless it is inserted very gently. Even then it may make the woman uncomfortable if it is introduced deeply. Joyful sex is very good for the muscles of the pelvic floor, and if you usually find complete relaxation difficult, note the full neuro-muscular release that comes after orgasm.

'FALSE' LABOUR AND PAINFUL BRAXTON-HICKS CONTRACTIONS

We don't know why the 'practice' contractions with which the uterus rehearses its role in labour – and which have persisted throughout pregnancy, although not all women are aware of them – may towards the end of pregnancy suddenly become not only much more noticeable but actually painful. However, a fair proportion of expectant mothers do experience painful Braxton-Hicks contractions during the last few weeks of pregnancy – some of the contractions may be so severe, rhythmical and recurrent that they feel sure labour is starting. Occasionally, the cervix is already partially dilated before a woman is aware she is in labour, and this may account for these contractions with some women. But the explanation for the majority must be sought in the psychological state of a woman who is approaching her expected date of birth – her excitement and anticipation, her longing to 'get on with it', her boredom and irritation with the long-continuing state of pregnancy, the knowledge that friends pregnant at the same time have already had their babies, and the feeling that with every day the baby is growing more and more enormous and more likely to involve a difficult labour the longer it is delayed. It is unwise to tell a woman that she 'may have it any day now', and particularly that she is having 'a big baby', since this adds to any latent anxiety – and at the back of the minds of many women is a longing for a small baby – even perhaps a little premature, because they think that labour may be easier.[3]

---

[3] A small baby does not necessarily mean a swift, easy labour, however, nor a large baby a painful and protracted one. A woman's preparation and emotional attitude are much more relevant factors.

HOW A MOTHER CAN HELP HER PREGNANT DAUGHTER

When a daughter is pregnant for the first time it is a problem for the mother to know how much advice she should give and how much she should try to enter into her daughter's life. She may be very thrilled, and usually is, about her daughter's pregnancy, and at the same time is a little anxious for her, worried that she may not be able to cope, perhaps with the pregnancy, perhaps also with the birth itself – and very probably with the new baby when it arrives.

Mothers want to share in their daughters' lives and are reminded vividly of the coming of their own first baby. Many daughters turn towards their mothers at this time, especially if there is a good relationship between them already.

But some daughters are still working through a stage of adolescent rebellion, a perfectly natural, almost inevitable stage, but one which can be very awkward and complicated for all concerned. We normally think of this stage as finishing at about the time a woman has a home of her own, if not before. But there are still a great many young women who are in a love–hate relationship with their mothers when they start their own families. This does not necessarily mean that they have cut loose from home and mother. Sometimes a woman is obviously dependent upon her mother – over-dependent – ringing her up or emailing her every day, consulting Mummy about everything. Mummy usually isn't worried about this sort of daughter; she ought to be of course, but 'smother mothers', who never managed to cut the emotional umbilical cord, really love their daughters to behave like this and encourage their overdependence. This sort of woman is in an infantile, preadolescent phase of relationship with her mother, and has somehow to mature before she can become a mother herself.

There is another sort of dependence not so worrying because it is an adolescent, not infantile, dependence. The younger woman appears not to care at all what her mother thinks and deliberately flouts her. But here too there is dependence upon her mother's values as all she is doing is consciously and deliberately rebelling against her mother's standards and ways of doing things instead of establishing her own independent set of values. She may seem very confident and self-assured, but is not.

A woman really does need her mother when she is pregnant, and has her first baby, but not for teaching her the right methods and ways of doing things, nor for taking over the baby when it arrives while the daughter has a nice rest, but for letting her see her approval of her daughter in her new role as a mother. Basically the grandmother's task is to look for what she can praise, and give her daughter the reassurance which can help her to build up her own image of herself as a mother.

Many grandmothers are not so good at this, partly because the methods and goals of childcare and running a house – and the partnership between the parents – are very different from what they were fifty years ago. The older generation of women were, on the whole, much more orderly and tidy. Their daughters' households look pretty chaotic to them. A grandmother may worry to see her daughter demand-feeding or cuddling her baby spontaneously, simply because he looks so delicious. She thinks that with no routine and by paying the baby 'unnecessary' attention, her daughter is merely making a rod for her own back. The grandmother may think back to her young days when mothers dared not move the infant till the clock struck the hour for feeds.

But there is more to it than that. Often the maternal grandmother longs to take over the child herself and show her daughter how it is all done. She probably sees it as protecting her. And just when her daughter needs reassurance that her baby is perfect – it is extremely common for mothers both during and after pregnancy to worry about their child's well-being – when the new mother is going through these frightening feelings of concern for the child and believing that she somehow cannot produce from her body something quite perfect, just then the grandmother asks worriedly, 'Do you think he's getting enough milk, dear? Don't you think your milk looks rather blue and watery?' or 'He isn't very fat, is he?' or 'Shouldn't she have a tooth by now?' These things are all said with the kindest of intentions, but emphasise the grandmother's lack of confidence in her daughter as a mother just when she needs her positive support and praise.

The grandmotherly interference can have an even greater impact during pregnancy, when the grandmother may suggest that her daughter's actions could endanger the baby's life or mar it in some way. One grandmother even admonished her daughter not to lift her arms above her head 'or the cord may get tangled around the baby's neck'. Such exaggerated concern serves only to alarm the younger woman.

Many women, especially when pregnant for the first time, feel a sense of guilt in relation to their own mothers. In some way they are replacing their mothers. They are the generation which is superseding their mothers as mothers. They often do not put this into words or even think about it, but they have the feeling that they are somehow, in some indefinable way, stealing something valuable from their mothers. It can come out into the open as a direct conflict for possession of the child, the grandmother wooing the child with sweets and presents and, the daughter says, spoiling him.

For it is not only daughters who lack confidence. Sometimes grandmothers lack confidence too. They want to know that they are loved. They want this child to demonstrate that he loves them; and if the grandmother's relationship with her own partner is not particularly happy and she does not feel valued for her own sake, she may attempt to get the love that she needs from her daughter's children.

The future grandmother who feels unloved and unwanted can make pregnancy a hard time for her daughter.

A first pregnancy can be a time of great stress anyway. To make this sometimes very difficult transition a woman has to be able to see herself as a mother and to *like* what she sees. A future grandmother does not need to ply her daughter with baby books and give a lot of advice. Girls acquire practical maternal skills most naturally and easily in childhood by example when they watch their mothers handling babies, whether they are their own brothers and sisters or relatives. Because they admire and love their mothers, they see her actions as admirable and then start to handle their dolls or animals or baby brothers and sisters in the same way, and to base their behaviour on their mother's. It is not really maternal instinct. It is *learned* behaviour, but learned mostly unconsciously, at an early age, when the small girl simply, naturally, as a part of her play, imitates her mother.

When the mother has been away because of illness, separation or divorce, and no one satisfactory has come to take her place, the younger woman has a much harder task. But even so any woman who can read and attend classes can learn all the practical details she needs to know about preparing for a baby just as she used her intelligence to learn the tasks she needed to know in order to hold down a job. It is a matter of getting the information.

However, the actual touch of a mother with her child does not come so easily if there has not been a mother or satisfactory mother-figure in one's own childhood. The touch of a mother with a newborn child is very different from that of one with a nine-month-old child or a two-year-old. It changes as the child gets older and is able to grow away from her a little bit and become more independent. And she does not have to stop to think about it. She feels the child's needs at that time and responds appropriately. Her touch, her gentle affectionate handling of her children, is one of the basic tenets of being a good mother. All other aspects of practical childcare – how to dress or bath the baby etc. – are superficial compared to how a mother instinctively touches her child. She does not need to analyse or question this innate skill – it would probably make her self-conscious and detract from her good instincts if she did. But in this field self-confidence is absolutely essential, and if the woman has not got self-confidence she pauses – she *does* stop and analyse the way to handle her baby, and then cannot relax and relate herself to the baby fully. So much that we think of as help for new mothers endangers this relationship. The preoccupation that a woman feels with her baby comes as near as possible to what it is to live in another person, and this is a very precious element in the baby's relationship with its mother at this stage of its life.

The most important – the essential – help and support that any grandmother can give to her daughter is to build up her confidence in herself, a feeling of rightness about being a mother and of the way she handles her baby, and to help her relate herself to the baby. If the daughter does not seem adult and capable of being an expert mother, there is even more reason for building up her self-confidence and giving her this loving support.

When a grandmother learns to do this she will have found a way for both mother and daughter to grow closer together as grown-up friends, in a new relationship that accepts that both are now adult. Only then can the new grandmother be of real help and contribute to her daughter's, and grandchild's, happiness.

BIRTH AS FULFILMENT

A woman can be happier when she is pregnant than at any other time in her life. It would give a very one-sided picture of pregnancy to concentrate exclusively on problems of adjustment and inner conflicts. She is often radiant with the new life within her, for which she has longed, even, perhaps, when they were taking precautions against conception.

To a man, having children is not an inherent part of sex. The baby does not grow in his body for nine long months, and the cleavage between the act of intercourse and the event of birth is complete for all but the most sensitive men who can imaginatively project themselves into a woman's feelings during pregnancy and childbirth. For a woman, longing for a child can be as disturbing and impelling as sexual desire alone can be for a man.

Probably few men even remember the nights on which their children were conceived. But women like to be able to think of that particular act of love as a special occasion memorable for the intensity of its passion and the depth of its tenderness. Sometimes if they are not sure when the baby was conceived they re-create the occasion in fantasy – from that precious moment the searching sperm entered deep into the woman and sought out the ovum in the darkness and warmth of her body.

Whatever minor discomforts may be involved in pregnancy, this time of preparation is for many women a very happy one, when they feel they are being used to the full, bear hope in their bodies despite all the cruelty and disaster of the world, and are sharing in the miracle of new life. During the first four months the baby does not seem a reality and a woman can hardly believe that she is pregnant, but once she feels quickening she begins to know and recognise her child and to form a relationship with it, even though the baby may prove rather different when born from what she expected. In the later months of pregnancy she conducts, as it were, a two-way conversation, with the world outside, and with the baby within her. She responds to communication coming from two different directions. As her body ripens and term approaches the reality of the experience which confronts her, and its inevitability, sometimes threatens her composure and she needs moral support from those who can describe birth as wonderful in itself, not just something to be lived through for the sake of having the baby. But the bravest of women approach it with something like timidity, even if it is a timidity born of awe rather than fear, for they are on the threshold of the unknown.

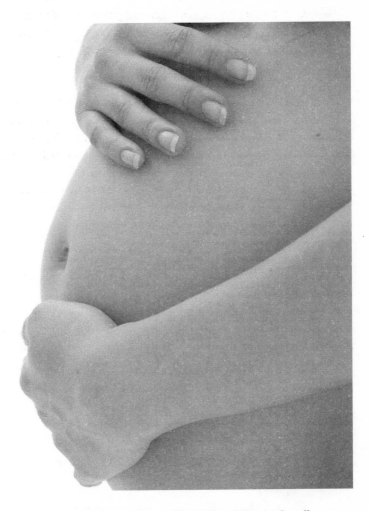

**Releasing all the muscles of the abdominal wall
enables breathing to be easy and full.**

5

Learning Harmony in Birth

The same stream of life that runs through my veins night and day runs through the world and dances in rhythmic measure. It is the same life that shoots in joy through the dust of the earth in numberless waves of grass and breaks into tumultuous waves of leaves and flowers. It is the same life that is rocked in the ocean-cradle of birth and of death, in ebb and in flow. I feel my limbs are made glorious by the touch of this world of life. And my pride is from the life-throb of ages dancing in my blood this moment.

Rabindranath Tagore, Gitanjali, lxix.

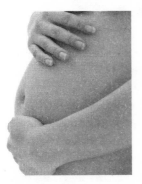

RELAXATION

The aim of the exercises described in the next three sections is to help a woman understand herself and her body better. None of the techniques are intended, for example, to be used to distract a woman from her labour. It is not a training aimed at occupying her mind with irrelevant physical activities to divert attention from sensations coming from the cervix. Every exercise she learns is designed to help her relate herself better to her body. She neither concentrates on a tune, in order not to 'notice' the intensity of the contraction, nor thinks of subjects far removed from the reality which she is experiencing, whether this is a sunny seashore or a diagram intended to represent a labour contraction (but which is, in fact, very far removed from anything a contraction *feels* like). There is nothing to escape from, nothing to deny, nothing she cannot face.

Nor is the aim simply a mechanical drill in which a woman says to herself, 'One, two, three, contract. One, two, three, relax.' Exercising at this level is probably not much help for labour. It is much more a question of what she thinks and feels about her body in relation to the tensions and the subsequent release from tension that she observes; a matter of the way she 'sees' her body. A French psychologist has said that 'relaxation is not simply learning at the level of muscular tone, but involves a maturing of the body image. In other words we simply cannot think of relaxation as a more or less specialised form of gymnastics, but must see it as an emotional experience involving a human being as an existential whole (embracing past, present and future).'[1]

Stanislavski, the great actor and producer, understood this. And in the acting system which he created he was concerned with developing outward action from what he called 'inner truth', from the very core of the person, the identity of each role that an actor must seek to understand and to interpret. For instance he said:

> In order to differentiate silk and velvet one needs another tempo and rhythm than in differentiating the bristles of a clothes brush. To smell ammonia one needs another tempo and rhythm than in smelling lilies of the valley. If one smells ammonia as one smells lilies of the valley, with rapid breathings-in of various duration and rhythm, one runs the risk of burning the whole mucous membrane of the nose. In a series of variegated exercises I tried to develop in my pupils not the outward rhythm of movement and action, but the inner rhythm of that unseen energy which calls out movement and action. In this manner I was able to develop in my pupils the sensation of movement and gesture, walking, and the entire inner pulse of life.[2]

In this chapter you will find a new approach to relaxation which, although it is based on Jacobson's teaching (see page 33), goes

---

[1] B. This, *Revue de Médecine psychosomatique*, vol 3, 2, 1961 (my translation).
[2] Constantin Stanislavski, *My Life in Art*, Bles, 1924.

beyond this and uses both techniques inspired by the Method School of acting and experiments in body-language and touch. This can be useful in coming to understand your body better as you are swept through the enormous physical and emotional changes of pregnancy, labour and motherhood. In becoming more aware of your relationship with your body you acquire a skill which helps you meet the challenge of birth, but, more than this – allows you to go *with* it, to surrender yourself to it, to answer the stimuli coming from your cervix with adaptive be-haviour of your whole body and your breathing rhythms. A 'muscle-bound' woman determined to do well, to put all she has learned into practice, to forget no part of her drill, is perhaps the one least likely to have a simple, smoothly functioning labour.

Becoming Aware of Relaxation and Tension in your Body

The ability to relax is not an inherent characteristic, born in some people but of which others are deprived. It can be acquired with practice and concentration, and some of those who think they are least able to relax and say that they never will be able to, relax better than those who face life generally with less apparent tension and who seem to have sleepier sorts of natures. Time and again I have seen emotionally taut, intelli-gent, self-critical and persevering women teach their bodies how to relax, controlling them with their minds, and develop-ing a skill which is useful not only in labour but whenever they find themselves tense in their daily lives.

Often in routine tasks about the home and office muscles are contracted unnecessarily and energy is wasted. If you observe yourself carefully when you are at the computer, beating eggs, polishing shoes, or even watching TV, you will probably dis-cover that you are tensing your shoulders, compressing your abdomen, gritting your teeth, holding your breath, or doing other things which give clear indication that you are not allow-ing your energy to flow naturally and easily into what you are doing. The first stage in learning relaxation is cultivating the ability to be aware of this.

Even so, some women protest that they cannot relax 'properly' – allow their minds to drift and be blank, and their bodies to sink into semi-slumber. You don't have to do this. Most of us lead lives that are too busy and have minds too active for trance-like relaxation.

If you feel wound up when you try to relax, use the activity of your mind to focus and concentrate upon control of specific muscles and groups of muscles. Think not in terms of passively submitting to a state of relaxation but of actively *stripping off tension*.

Exercise 1

Lie down comfortably, head and shoulders raised and firmly supported, with all joints well flexed and plenty of cushions wherever you want them, in a warm but airy room,[3] and close your eyes. Feel them heavy lidded. Feel the whole eye as heavy. Listen to the sound of your breathing, and with each breath out concentrate on stripping off muscular tension wherever you are aware of it. Feel your shoulder-blades as if they were opening outwards, like a dress that is slipping off a hanger at both ends. Contract your abdominal muscles and then feel the easy release as you relax them. Feel your chest tight all round, and then consciously release those muscles so that it expands loosely with each breath out. Breathe in and out for a little while like this until you are quite sure that your breathing is effortless and full.

Now make the breath out a little longer – as long as you can comfortably make it. Breathe in through your nose and out through your mouth, emphasising the breath out and relaxing a little more with each breath out; let the breath in look after itself. Feel as if you are breathing right down your back. If you have good back support, all the way up from the bottom of your spine to the top of your head, which includes support in the small of the back and behind the neck, you will feel a slight, almost imperceptible movement along the length of the spine as you breathe. After all, it is constructed more like a string of sausages than a lamp-post. Breathe steadily and rhythmically and

---

[3] A cold atmosphere makes muscles contract.

note that faint movement of the vertebrae as you continue breathing in and out. Use your breathing to relax further.

Are there any points at which you are still tense? You will help yourself if you can think of them as warm, as if you have just had a hot water bottle there. If this is insufficient a hot water bottle (not too hot) actually resting behind your shoulders or between your legs or wherever it is that you are still tense will help. Once you have got the idea of feeling muscles warm you will be able to *imagine* them warm and so release them consciously. Feel your scalp warm as if you have just come out from under a hair dryer, warm and tingling.

Feel each limb heavy, every bone heavy, the pull of gravity drawing your body down to the earth. Allow your knees to flop apart, your whole body to feel as if it is melting.

All this is much easier if your partner, or a friend with whom you do not feel self-conscious, reads the exercise instructions out aloud to you once you have had an initial try yourself in privacy, and tests your relaxation as you proceed. It is reassuring to know that you really are achieving something, and only too easy to think that you are relaxed when, in fact, you are very far from it. Your partner can pick up a hand and let it drop, noting if there is any resistance, smoothly and slowly move your hand in circles from the wrist, your arm at the elbow, and, holding your hand, your arm at the shoulder, to feel whether any of the works need oiling. A helper who is tempted to criticise your performance or to get impatient can try relaxing. It is not so easy. Criticism should always be positive and constructive. After the hand and arm, he tests your legs. First with a hand under the ankle he lifts the leg from the knee and lets it drop. Then, once there is no resistance, your partner bends one leg so that the knee is raised towards the abdomen, and then moved in a circle. Make sure that the muscle running along the inside of the upper leg, the adductor, is well released, or this can be uncomfortable.

If you are lying with your head fairly low and really well relaxed your helper can hold your toes and shake them firmly and gently, and you will shake all the way up to your head, which wobbles on top like one of those Japanese wooden dolls. (Of course all this is slightly ridiculous and I hope that you will find yourselves laughing about it. It should not be taken dead seriously. Laughter helps you to relax.)

Your partner rests a hand on either side of the pelvis, low on your hips, and gently and firmly rocks you from side to side. Then he holds your head in his hands and does the same, lifting your chin up and down and rocking your head also towards the chest and up again. You feel your head warm and heavy, like a great ball.

When you get up after lying relaxed always have a good stretch and see if you can make yourself yawn. Get up slowly, gradually unfolding, like Cleopatra rising from her barge, if you can conjure up this image in pregnancy! If you jump straight up you may feel giddy.

Exercise 2

Start with the first exercise and then discover the points at which you personally are liable to have unnecessary tension.

When you are well relaxed begin to think especially about the muscles of your face. Our moods and thoughts are quickly reflected in our faces. Every muscle can respond to the emotions of joy, grief, tenderness, love or hate.

Concentrate first on the cheeks. Feel them warm and rosy. As you breathe in, allow your nostrils to dilate slightly, and let the breathing movement spread across your cheeks. Let your lips part slightly, smooth and soft, as if you have just put on a new and expensive lipstick! The tip of your tongue rests against the inside of your front lower teeth. The tongue is broad and soft.

Your jaw is relaxed; let it go at the point where it joins the skull just in front of your ears. Think of your eyelids as heavy. Feel the space between the eyes getting wider and wider. Your brow is smooth and broad. Your face is now relaxed.

Stanislavski Relaxation

These imaginative exercises grew out of Stanislavski acting techniques. They are based on the Method School of acting, and I have devised them from my own acting training many years ago.

Start by thinking of your eyes. Do you know when they are really relaxed? Close them and do the following exercises:

Exercise 1

Imagine there is a ship sailing away from you and you are watching it move towards the distant horizon. Follow its course carefully; keep your eyes on it. As it approaches the horizon your eyes are in a more relaxed state than when you were focusing on it close up. Then rest your eyes and you will realise that now the ship has disappeared entirely they are still more relaxed.

Exercise 2

Imagine that you have a newspaper in front of you with a photograph of the Queen. Focus your eyes firmly on it. Then relax. Now spread out this imaginary newspaper and start to read it, and you will feel the pull of your eye muscles from left to right and back to the beginning of the line. Relax.

Exercise 3

See a large six-storey building in front of you and watch a firefighter hoist a ladder and climb slowly up to the top. You will feel a different muscular pull as your eyes move in a different direction. Now watch him slowly coming down again. He is at the bottom. Rest your eyes.

Exercise 4

You are watching a tennis match. Feel the muscle tension as you keep your eye on the ball. Now rest your eyes and you will experience a release from tension which is very pleasant.

'See' mentally a vivid scarlet, green and white detergent advertisement just in front of you. Look far into the distance at blue-hazed mountains, very still in the morning air. You will experience a feeling of relief as the strain on the eyes disappears.

You can do these exercises with your eyes open, too.

Exercise 5

Now get into a position in which you can move your arms and imagine that you are carrying a large and heavy, precious crystal bowl. Feel it in your hands as you mime the movement. The tension will also be felt in your arms and shoulders and in your eyes, since you must watch it. Then put it down, and relax.

Exercise 6

Concentrate on imaginatively walking along a thin white line, one foot carefully in front of the other. You will feel tension in the arch of your feet, toes, thighs, buttocks and lower back, and also in your arms, hands and shoulders as you strive to keep your balance. Now step off the line and relax completely.

Exercise 7

Imagine that you are getting into very cold water, toes first; sink right under gradually, feeling the icy water rise up your back and over you, and then get out and throw yourself on a warm beach in the sun. Feel the sand hot under your body, the sun pouring into your skin with the warm air on the surface of your skin. Visualise yourself falling into a deep, restful sleep lying there. Stand outside yourself, as it were, and see your body lying there in the hot sunlight, breathing peacefully, perfectly relaxed.

Exercise 8

You are driving a car. Imagine that you are about to overtake, and notice another car overtaking and coming towards you on the wrong side of the road. Observe the tensions that result in your eyes, arms, shoulders, and the leg with which you step on the brake. Now feel this tension 'uncoil', and relax completely.

Exercise 9

Imagine that you are stooping down to get a dish out of the oven. Feel the contraction of your muscles as you imagine bending; turn the handle of the oven door; move a little away as the heat comes into your face, and then, carefully holding an oven cloth, lean forward and take the heavy casserole out. You will be aware of a whole series of different kinds of tensions in these often repeated movements, involving muscles in your back, feet and legs, your hands, neck, face and arms. Now let all this tension go, and relax again.

You can invent imaginary activities for yourself in this way, and observe the tensions that each involves.

Inventing your own Exercises

Once you have reached this stage of learning relaxation – and not only relaxation, but a much more intricate and subtle awareness of your body – you are ready to start using your imagination and ability to remember patterns of contractions in different everyday situations involving stress, to evolve exercises of your own based on the tensions which you personally are inclined to have. That is, you start with simple actions, as when you pull open a heavy drawer which has stuck, push a door which has caught on the carpet, or open a door with one hand whilst balancing a tray in the other. Having observed and isolated them, the next task is to re-create these particular contractions, as you lie down practising your relaxation. They can even be done in the bath. Always relax between the actions or you may find that you carry over residual tension from the last one.

Here are a few suggestions, to which you will be able to add many:

1. You have a mouth full of neat lemon juice. Relax.
2. You are breathing in the fumes from an open bottle of ammonia. Relax. It is gone!
3. You are walking on the beach, barefoot, with sharp, jagged pebbles under your feet. Pick your way carefully up the beach. Then relax.

From there, move on to situations of stress involving emotional conflict. Here you begin to draw on your personal experience of life - tensions which, perhaps, nobody else is aware of. Try to be honest with yourself and to note and analyse the tensions carefully. None of us goes through life cool, calm and collected all of the time. In a book I can only throw out a few hints and suggestions, basing these on tensions many women experience.

Do not attempt to re-create an emotion in yourself without re-creating the *specific circumstances* which lead up to the expression of this emotion, or what you do will be forced and artificial. 'Don't think about the feeling itself, but set your mind to work on what makes it grow, what the conditions were that brought about the experience . . . *Never begin with results. They will appear in time as the logical outcome of what has gone before.*'[4]

1. You are whisking cream in a hurry, with a rather elegant guest just about to come into the kitchen.
2. You are waiting at the booking-office for your ticket and the train is just about to leave.
3. Walking down a lonely country lane at night (it is pitch dark) you think you hear someone walking behind you. He seems to be creeping in the shadow of the hedge. Did you hear a noise? Notice your reactions. How was your breathing affected?
4. You are in a public place, feeling very upset and desperately wanting to cry but not wanting anyone to see how unhappy you are. Notice the tightness of your face – like a mask – the tensed abdominal muscles, the dry feeling in the throat, and the effect on your breathing. What other muscles are contracted?

Now concentrate on situations and things that you really worry about or fear. Sometimes these fears are irrational, occasionally reasonable. Make a list (you can burn it afterwards) of those subjects which involve great stress, which worry you deeply, or of which you are afraid. Include anything to do with your baby, pregnancy, the hospital, your relationships, or the way your body works. Perhaps the list is small – do not artificially manufacture fears – but it will still provide material for practice.

1. Select one subject and give your imagination free rein so that it is vivid and real for you to work on. You are going to relive the tensions associated with it, whether it is a mouse running along the floor, someone staying in the house who causes unhappiness, your toddler almost knocked down by a car, the empty house at night with the door creaking, or things like the pain of a menstrual period or a miscarriage, being constipated, an asthma attack or migraine, or even

---

[4] Constantin Stanislavski, *An Actor Prepares*, Bles, 1937.

having a tooth drilled at the dentist's (but in this case start off analysing your tensions in the waiting-room).

2. Imagine yourself looking out over the edge of a high building, or shut in a cupboard under the stairs or a lift which has stuck. Think of a situation in which you have become so worked up that you felt like bursting with rage – those few seconds before you struck out or screamed or fled. Think perhaps of a particularly unpleasant dream that has been haunting you – the knife edge, the locked cupboard or narrow passage, squirming snakes or crawling insects, being tied down on an operating table, on the edge of a precipice or drowning. Most women seem to have intensified and often uncomfortable dreams in pregnancy. Really act it, and once you are living the part, stand outside yourself and observe yourself in it. What muscles are contracted? How are you breathing? Where is the tension concentrated?

Now consciously, deliberately, send a message from your brain to the muscles involved – rather like a telephone message – switching the contractions off. Relax completely.

Summon up the picture again, repeat the exercise. Switch off the contractions instantaneously when you wish to relax.

Summon up the picture again, and this time *meet* it with relaxation instead of tension. This may be difficult at first. You will acquire skill as you practise.

Gradually you will develop a new neuro-muscular awareness – quite different from intellectual knowledge about your body. It will be useful to you not only in labour, but in every situation to which you react with tension – and is a firm basis on which to build relaxation for labour. Controlled relaxation derived from an understanding of yourself and your personal reactions is the starting point. When you have achieved this you are already halfway along the road.

Touch Relaxation

Another approach to relaxation can be made through touch and, best of all, the touch of someone you love. The following exercises are designed to increase awareness of body tensions and release, and also to be a pleasure in themselves. They can be done in bed, and preferably with no or few clothes on. This method can be useful if you find the imaginative exercises we have just been doing difficult because you seem unable to visualise the situations easily. But ideally, try different approaches to relaxation and aim at being expert with them all.

The aim of touch relaxation is to by-pass words and try to use other forms of stimulus. To do this we aim at building up non-verbal communication based on touch.

Not everyone relaxes in response to the same sort of stimulus and methods of teaching relaxation ought to be as varied as the women to whom we try to teach them. In my own teaching of relaxation I have found it useful to experiment with a wide range of verbal imagery, and to attempt all the time to adapt my teaching to what appear to me to be the needs of each particular woman. Even the best image may fail dismally for a woman with whom, because of her personal experience and memories, the words conjure up a situation which is either unknown, or preposterous, or uncomfortable. A few pages back I suggested that complete release of muscles of the scalp felt as if your head was warm – as if you had just come out from under the hair dryer. When I once mentioned this to a student she flinched at the thought, and protested, 'But I can't *bear* that! I *hate* that feeling!'

So we need not depend upon verbal stimuli alone. Our culture is, or has been up till now, a highly verbal one, and we tend to teach through and with words when sometimes there are other means of communication open to us – which we need not leave to chance or spontaneous impulse – such as when we smile or lean forward, or reach out a hand.

Non-verbal communication, which is taking place all the time alongside verbal methods, and which may intrude on and actually alter the message of verbal communication, can itself be examined, analysed and structured so that we can use it deliberately, with forethought and skill.

I suggest using non-verbal communication as one way of achieving neuro-muscular release, and find this simplest to base on the spontaneous way in which a couple touch each other, because they like to, and because it gives them pleasure, comfort, reassurance, erotic delight and companionship. I have an abhorrence of the sort of antenatal exercise which entails putting on leotards and leaping around doing a parade-ground drill for 'B day', and although I realise that some women find it very cheering I cannot see how, apart from pepping up the circulation, it can have any possible influence on a woman's effective adaptive responses in childbirth.

But labour, anyway, is not the be-all-and-end-all of life, and to practise only with the few hours of labour in mind is to limit our skill in relaxation unnecessarily. After the birth, what then? The woman is holding a baby in her arms. And how does she hold it? When she is feeding the baby, and changing it and bathing it, and when she holds her toddler, or copes in the kitchen or does her housework, writes her thesis, or deals with illness in the family, when she is driving a car, or shopping, or offering help to someone in distress, or dealing with all the maddening, chaotic, nerve-racking, ear-splitting crises in a family . . . how is she then? Of course the answer is that we scream and weep; and we get headaches and all sorts of psychosomatic illnesses, and we say things we wish to heaven we hadn't said, and then we feel guilty because we have done all these things; we make valiant efforts to improve – prayer or meditation over the washing-up perhaps, and earnest discussion with other equally guilty mums. This is how I am anyway, and it is because I know my own besetting sins that I feel relaxation should be tackled at the level of ordinary, everyday living and be something helpfully de-stressing that we can incorporate into life.

The basic grammar of this non-verbal language of touch is simple – release *flowing out towards* the touching hand; this is what you do spontaneously when someone you love touches you. At the same time it is important that your partner learns to touch with a relaxed hand, slowly, moulding the hand to the shape of the limb or any other part of the body on which the couple is working. Thus it is a mutual exercise in release, and there is never a question of the pregnant woman becoming a criticised pupil. Instead they are participating together in what is really not so much an exercise as a 'sensitivity response'.

You contract a set of muscles, and when you are ready your partner rests a hand on the contracted muscles. The moment this happens, release towards the hand. There are various ways in which this can be done, and it is a good idea to concentrate on parts of the body which you find it difficult to relax. Lie on your back, propped up and well supported with pillows in a warm bed, with support all up your spine, including the small of your back and the back of your neck, and under your knees. Breathe out and relax completely. The following are ways of exploring ease of release over different parts of the body:

1. Frown. Your helper rests a hand on your brow. Relax.
2. Grit your teeth and clench your jaw. The helper rests a hand on either side of your jaw. Relax.
3. Contract muscles of the scalp and raise your eyebrows. Your partner rests hands on either side of the scalp. Relax.
4. Press your shoulder-blades back as if they were angel's wings and you could make them touch each other. Your partner rests a hand at the front of each shoulder. Relax.
5. Pull in your abdominal wall towards your spine. The helper rests both hands on the lower curve of your abdomen. Relax.
6. Press your upper legs together as if you could hold a sheet of paper between them. The partner touches the outside of each leg. Relax and your legs flop apart.
7. Press your legs out, still flexed, but forcing your thighs apart. Your partner rests a hand on the inside of each thigh. Relax.
8. Contract the muscles of your right arm like a wooden doll, with fingers stretched out, but without raising it. Your partner first rests both hands firmly on your shoulder and inner upper arm and you relax. Then slowly, with one hand still on the shoulder, your helper runs the other hand down the arm on the inside to the waist, and you relax still further. Repeat with the other arm.
9. Contract the muscles of one leg by pointing your toes up towards the ceiling and straightening your leg (not if it causes cramp). Your helper places one hand over the inside upper leg and the other over the outside, moulding both

hands to the shape of your body. Relax your whole leg. Then, slowly and deliberately, in one long stroke, your partner moves both hands down the leg to the ankle, finishing with one hand holding your bare foot firmly round the instep. (If this is not done firmly it will tickle you.) This slow movement helps you let any residual tension flow out, as if into the cradling hands. Repeat with the other leg.

Then turn on your side or in the front lateral – three-quarters over with your upper knee drawn up near your breast – whichever is the most comfortable, and in this position:

10. Raise your chin in the air and contract muscles at the back of your neck. Your helper rests a hand in the nape of your neck and you release.

11. Hollow the small of your back. Your helper rests both hands against either side of the sacro-lumbar spine and you release.

12. Press your buttocks together. Your partner rests a hand on each buttock, and you relax.

Each of these tensions is related to common stress situations to which we tend to react with tension, both in everyday life, and in different phases of labour.

We often contract muscles of the scalp and back of the neck – as in Exercise 3, for instance – when we have a headache, and sometimes contraction of these muscles in situations of stress precedes the onset of a tension headache, and might be the cause of the pain. In Exercise 4, contraction of muscles of the shoulders and the top of the back are involved, in just the way that they may be when there is a build-up of tension in the late first stage of labour. Contraction of these muscles is very likely to result in over-breathing and consequent hyperventilation of the maternal bloodstream, which we shall see more about when we discuss breathing in labour. The initial effect is to make breathing more difficult; it becomes forced and hectic, and light, easy breathing gives way to heavy panting. The cause is not so much that the breathing is wrong, but that the woman has become tense and is no longer able to breathe gently.

In Exercise 8 you get an idea of the help a partner can give simply by touch, using a hand to help you relax, and this is better than encouraging you to cling on to the hand. For this reason it is a good idea during contractions to hold you by the wrist rather than grip your hand, and then to stroke the muscles of the arm down from the shoulder to help remind you of the need for complete release.

Exercise 9 gives an idea of tension that can build up in transition, the difficulty in relaxing which a woman may encounter when her legs get extremely cold and start to shake, as they often do just at the onset of the second stage before she begins pushing, and how she can consciously and carefully relax them.

Exercise 10 depicts the woman who in the second stage bears down using her throat muscles and strains excessively in a frantic effort to push the baby out. This can be corrected in the same way as in the second part of the exercise, by firm touch at the back of the neck which reminds her to release her neck muscles and let her chin drop forward on to her chest.

It is during the expulsive stage that many women feel despair, unable to make headway, and start to contract muscles in the back, lifting the small of the back away from the delivery table or bed. This again can be corrected with firm pressure of the partner's hand against this part of her back.

In Exercises 11 and 12 we get a picture of a woman who is resisting the odd sensations of pressure. This can make her feel as if the baby is coming out of the 'wrong hole' and that she is going to pop. The fetal head descends through the birth canal, feels as if it fills the rectum and anus, and later spreads open the vagina. Both the adductors inside the upper legs, and *glutei*, or buttock muscles, may contract if she is fighting these sensations.

So touch relaxation techniques can also find a place in labour, and are a valuable means of offering practical support, which neither involves nagging nor puts you in the situation where you feel: 'Who's having this baby – you or me?'

The companion who is alert and sensitive to the build-up of tension, however slight, can rest a hand on muscles involved, both between contractions, and, if you wish, at the onset of contractions.

Sometimes a woman does not like being touched at all during labour and wants to be left alone because she finds contact irritating. Each couple must work out what is best for them and what they personally want to do at that time. A birth companion needs to be sensitive, since touch can also be an intrusion, and should only be used in labour when you find it really helpful.

Relaxing in Childbirth

Every time a muscle contracts there is a shortening and drawing-up of muscle fibre.

During the first stage of labour, when the slow dilatation of the cervix is taking place, all those muscles which can be controlled by the brain should be relaxed so that the muscles of the uterus which are pulling up the opening can work undisturbed. When you are relaxed, you begin to feel as if your body is spreading sideways and flowing out of its boundaries, rather like a very ripe Camembert!

Relaxation can be practised once or twice a day for ten minutes or so at a time, and on going to bed at night, when it will help to ensure sound, restful sleep. Use this time to think about being in labour, visualise the physiological processes during the first and second stages, and look forward to the experience.

After each period of neuro-muscular release stretch fully once or twice, like a cat in front of a fire, letting energy flow through all your muscles, yawn widely with a deep breath in and a long sigh out, and then get up slowly. In this way you will not only avoid any giddiness from moving too suddenly but will feel refreshed and reinvigorated.

Practise relaxation in different positions. Although you may like relaxing in the front lateral position and lying, head and shoulders propped, on your back with your knees drawn up, it is important to be able to relax in any position in which you may find yourself when in labour.

If you are going by car to hospital practise relaxation in the car. I know one woman who drove to hospital on the back of a motor-bike, relaxing well whilst using sufficient muscular tension to sit firmly on the machine and not fall off. One woman who came to my classes was a pilot, and flew up till the day her baby was born. She practised relaxation in the small space afforded in the cockpit, just in case she should start labour when in the air.

If labour is fast you may find that you are busy getting things ready at a point when you must concentrate on contractions and break off your activity to cope with them. It is helpful to be able to relax while standing. Some women lean slightly forward with their legs apart, their elbows resting on a shelf or table, and feel the lower part of the body go limp. Others like to lean forward with the fingertips resting on a piece of furniture. Some sway slightly forward and backward with a rocking movement of the pelvis during contractions in this position. Some like to squat down with the pelvis at its widest. Whatever positions you choose, there is no hard-and-fast rule about what you should do. The positions and movements in which you are most comfortable are right for you.

The relaxation needed in labour is the kind required to do any sport, to dance, play the piano, drive a car or ride a bicycle. All unnecessary tension is eliminated, everything that is not required for the task in hand. You do not collapse in a heap on the floor or render yourself unconscious to your environment, going into a trance and out of touch with those who are there to help. You are fully aware of all that is going on, mentally alert and in control of the situation. As each contraction comes, you begin the rhythmic, controlled breathing that enables you to keep abreast of your labour, and enjoy its excitement and the energy released in your body.

Massage

Massage is most effective when it is rehearsed before the birth by you and your birth partner. The first thing to remember is that all the massage for labour should be done with a relaxed hand and you always relax *towards* the massaging hands, so this help becomes a joint activity and not something to which you passively submit. You can use body lotion if you wish. If the other person wears a wedding ring it should be removed or it will feel like knuckledusters.

It may be useful to practise these seven types:

1. *Massage of the sacro-lumbar region.* Lie in the front lateral position (three-quarters over) or on your side. A firm hand is needed, curved to the shape of the small of the back, with pressure on the heel of the hand. It is best done so that the flesh moves over the bone, and is least effective when the hand just makes a slippery, stroking movement over a wide area. Every now and again the hand is swept down over the sides of your pelvis and over your buttocks. Slightly press the small of your back towards the hand.

2. *Whole back massage.* Kneel or lie in any position in which your partner can reach your back. Both hands are used to do long, firm stroking movements from your shoulders right down the back and around the curve of the buttocks. The hands are rested either side of the spine and flow in a continuous, but *slow*, movement, one hand on the lower back while the other is just starting at the shoulders.

3. *Kneading the buttocks.* Anyone who has ever made bread without a bread machine will know how to do this one! It consists of firm massage over the buttock muscles with a slow, leisurely movement, and is useful when the baby is pressing low against the rectum to ensure complete release of those muscles of the pelvic floor which are around the anus. Release towards the touch.

4. *Upper back massage.* Although the baby is going to emerge from the other end, it is often surprising how firm rubbing of the area around the shoulders can help you relax and keep your breathing rhythmic and unstrained. Here again, release towards the massaging hand.

5. *Massage of the adductors.* Facing you, the partner massages the muscles of the inner thigh from perineum to knee firmly and rhythmically, every now and again sweeping a hand over the outside of your thighs. Sit or lie on your back, legs flopped apart, knees out, and release your muscles consciously *towards* your partner, *including the muscles of the pelvic floor.*

In labour, as the contraction starts, your partner begins firm regular massage of the adductors. This is a highly effective way of gaining control even after it has been lost for a few contractions, and can be extremely useful at the end of the first stage and during transition (the bridge between the first and second stages).

6. *Light abdominal massage.* Many women find it comforting to stroke the area above the dilating cervix during contractions, and this can be done by the partner, too, with a very light touch. It is best done as if gently stroking the baby's head, curving from one side, down towards the pubis, and then up again a little at the other side, with one hand following on the other in a continuous stroking movement.

7. *Foot holding.* Some women appreciate firm holding of the balls of the feet with both hands, pressure being applied by the thumbs just at the top centre of the curve of the insteps. It is worth experimenting to find what feels good. Since these are acupuncture points which relate to the solar plexus, this is most likely to be useful during difficult contractions which threaten to 'take your breath away', to help keep your breathing rhythmic.

What's Going on in your Head?

Just as – if not more – important than what you are doing with your body is what is happening in your thinking. This is where creative fantasy and imagery help. You can prepare yourself to visualise the power of contractions sweeping through you and opening your cervix as the baby is descending, turning its head, and pressing down.

If your mind is distracted because you are angry or frustrated with yourself or anyone else, if you are preoccupied with being caught in cross-fire between people who are with you, or feel you have to fight a running battle with your care-givers, this mental restlessness blurs the positive focus on the work that your body is doing. You lose the tune. You miss steps in the dance.

In some Mediterranean and Indian birth cultures a flower is

placed near the labouring woman and she knows that as the petals open and spread out, her body is opening too. In some European traditional cultures, in peasant Greece, for example, the midwife and the helping women would undo all knots, unbutton the father's shirt, and make the way free symbolically for the baby to be born. Choose an image that enables you to relax, open and give. It need not be visual. It could be music that builds up in a grand crescendo, or kinetic – skiing, swimming over waves, or climbing a mountain.

Try this imagery exercise. Run a warm bath, shake in some drops of pure lavender oil. Light aromatic candles in the bathroom and play relaxing music or ocean wave sounds. As you lie in the water picture yourself in labour, waves of energy sweeping through your uterus, the cervix soft and opening, your baby curled up with its chin on its chest and pressing down . . . and down . . . and down, and all the soft tissues of your vagina fanning out and spreading wide.

BREATHING

It might be thought that we could safely leave breathing to chance, and that most women in labour breathe all right anyway. But women in labour frequently flush out too much carbon dioxide from their bloodstream with a resulting reduction in the flow of blood to the baby. Nor does training for birth avoid this problem if they are taught to pant heavily, and do deep, quick breathing, or when they are actually in labour if they start to gasp and 'huff and puff'. So it is important not only to learn how to breathe in an easy, relaxed, rhythmic way, but to *allow for a margin of error* in the stress of labour, particularly near full dilatation. The way you breathe is closely connected with the rhythm to which your body adapts itself in labour. If you can harmonise your breathing with the contractions of the uterus, which have a rhythm of their own and are like waves in the way that they gather, rise to a crest, and then die away, you will find it very exhilarating.

Before a woman has a baby she may think that birth entails

a great deal of pushing and straining and that the really important purpose of exercises is to develop very strong abdominal
muscles. But it is more a matter of breathing and co-ordination
than of straining and making terrific muscular efforts to expel
the baby.

Many women find the harmony they create between the
contractions and their breathing is exhilarating. It is similar
to the way in which smooth co-ordination of breathing and
muscular activity brings pleasure to a skilled runner. The sense
of well-being that results testifies to the release of endorphins
in the bloodstream that not only reduce or eradicate pain, but
produce elation. Even when contractions are very fierce – at the
end of the first stage of labour when the cervix is almost fully
dilated – by synchronising breathing with the rhythm of the
contractions it is possible for labour to be pleasurable, like
swimming in a stormy sea.

If a woman tries to resist the contractions, or merely to
endure them, she will have severe pain; instead, she needs to
go *with* them to get her baby born. So, as each one comes, *greet
it with your breathing*.

Rhythmic breathing ensures adequate oxygenation in both
pregnancy and labour. Many women habitually breathe very
shallowly, with only the top half of their chests. The baby re-
ceives oxygen from the mother's blood supply. *She breathes for
her baby*. When we engage in strenuous activity, or any muscle is
contracting hard, oxygen is used up more rapidly. When the
uterus is contracting in labour its extraordinary activity can use
up much of the oxygen in the bloodstream, and an accumula-
tion of toxic substances in turn can result in the pain of cramp.

Apart from its direct effect upon the uterus, shortage of
oxygen may also lead to quickening of the pulse, breathlessness,
and exhaustion.

As labour contractions become very forceful at the end of
the first stage a woman usually finds it easier to breathe more
shallowly and more lightly than she did earlier in labour, and
this often occurs spontaneously. But this lighter breathing can
lead to an inadequate oxygen supply if she starts gasping and
holding her breath in pain. She has to learn to breathe both

shallowly and *rhythmically*, and to breathe out deeply at the end of each contraction to compensate for the shallowness of the breathing during the contraction.

Rhythmic breathing can also help because it is almost impossible to panic when breathing carefully and concentrating on it. So closely is breathing connected with emotions that the first signs of fear, frustration, or anger are registered in a changed respiratory rhythm, and just as emotions affect your breathing, so it can work the other way and breathing steadily and carefully can keep you calm and tranquil. You may have noticed the change in rhythm and the deeper, slower breathing you tend to use when concentrating hard on something, the quicker, shallower breathing when you are excited or anticipating something exciting, the irregular arhythmic breathing of surprise.

Concentrating on the breathing rhythm also has the effect of centring the woman's attention on something she can actively do to help herself, so that she does not suffer labour passively, but engages positively in adjustment to what is happening in her body. The mind – not only the uterus – is an important factor in birth.

Breathing easily probably also helps to alleviate discomfort and pain by preventing unnecessary pressure on the abdomen.

The Diaphragm

Your diaphragm is attached to the inside of your lower ribs. Immediately above it and inside the cage of the thorax are the bottle-shaped lungs. As you breathe in, the diaphragm falls, flattens itself and spreads out, at the same time rising slightly at the edges, and your ribs are lifted by the intercostal muscles and spread out. As they do this, extra space is created in your thorax and you can fill your lungs with fresh air. When you breathe out again the diaphragm relaxes and stale air is released, but there is some residual air left in your lungs. When you have breathed out naturally and without strain, extra air can always be exhaled by using the muscles of your abdomen, which are also attached to the lower ribs. As you exert a strong pull on your abdominal muscles by pressing them in, your lungs are compressed so that carbon dioxide is forced out. The abdominal muscles used in this way terminate the respiratory activity which has been begun by the diaphragm.

From the sixth to seventh months of pregnancy the fundus of the uterus is much nearer the diaphragm, and each time a woman breathes in the diaphragm is pressed down towards it. This can make breathing rather difficult until the time when the baby 'drops' or 'lightens' and there is more space around the middle. The obstetric term for this is engagement and it usually occurs any time after about six weeks before the baby is due in a woman having her first baby – but often not till nearer the expected date of birth with a woman having her second or later babies.

The Abdominal Muscles

Your abdominal muscles are not consciously used in normal relaxed breathing. This happens only with powerful deep breathing such as may be used in voice production, in verse speaking, drama and singing. They do not need to be used consciously in labour either. The pressure of the abdominal muscles on the contracting uterus at the height of the first stage can be very uncomfortable, since it is acutely sensitive to pressure.

At first sight it seems strange that merely tightening the abdominal wall could cause pain. The movement of the abdominal wall in respiration is so obviously less drastic in its effects than the great waves of contraction undergone by the uterus. But the acute sensitivity of the uterus and surrounding layers of abdominal muscle to pressure during labour can be experienced during an otherwise painless contraction by simply strongly tensing your abdominal muscles at the height of a contraction. Women usually find palpation of the uterus during a contraction also very painful, and midwives should avoid this. It used to be suggested by some of the first exponents of 'natural' or prepared methods of childbirth in Britain (notably Minnie Randall[5] and Dr Kathleen Vaughan[6]) that steady pressure of the

---

[5] Minnie Randall, *Training for Childbirth*, Churchill, 1949.
[6] Kathleen Vaughan, *Safe Childbirth*, Baillière, 1937.

abdominal muscles during a contraction would speed up and ease the pains of labour by guiding the baby's head down into the pelvis and the birth canal. Those women who tried it may have experienced unnecessary pain.

Obstetric physiotherapists who followed Helen Heardman's teachings believed that a tense abdominal wall would cause pain by pressure on the uterus. So women were advised to breathe slowly in for fifteen seconds and slowly out for fifteen seconds, allowing the abdominal wall to expand with inhalation and to sink back with exhalation. But a woman may not be able to move her abdominal wall at all once the first stage is well under way.

The answer, I believe, is that the abdominal muscles can be released from tension and the pain of labour reduced or even wiped out by *releasing the abdominal wall completely* – that is, by allowing it to rest, carefully avoiding, on the one hand, trying to keep it still and, on the other, forcible movement of the abdominal wall when breathing, both of which can lead to excessive pain.

Relaxation of the Abdominal Muscles

Some women find relaxation of the abdominal wall difficult, especially when they are in any pain. They have been taught to 'hold their tummies in', and sometimes it runs against the grain to release these muscles. If a woman finds it does not come easily she must first be more aware of what contraction of these muscles feels like. Only by doing the opposite to relaxation and by studying the movements associated with contraction of these muscles can she learn how to let them 'give'.

Exercise 1

Lie on your back on the floor or on a firm bed, head raised on pillows, legs together. Relax. Now imagine that you are pulling over your hips some jeans that are much too tight for you. Pull them on a bit further, and then further still. Now you have to do up the zip at the side. Then relax completely. You will feel as if the tension is 'peeled off' from the muscles.

Exercise 2

In the same position, rest your fingers on your abdomen and lift your head to look at your toes. Immediately you feel the pull of these abdominal muscles. Lie flat again and stretch right down one side; you will feel the pull of the lower abdominal muscles and all the muscles along that side of the abdomen. Now do the same with the other leg. Then bend your knees and relax, letting the abdominal wall go.

Exercise 3

Now imagine that you are blowing on a candle flame in front of your pursed lips. Bend the flame only, and blow on it with steady pressure without putting it out. To get the added control required for this you find that you are automatically using the pressure of the abdominal muscles. You feel them pulling just below the ribs, across the waistline and spreading out.

Exercise 4

Once you are sure of the action of the abdominal muscles as you do these exercises, start to study the more subtle action of the diaphragm. One way is to breathe in fully and then breathe out in short, sharp rapid breaths, as if you were panting after running fast. You will feel the diaphragm moving as you do this. When you do the candle-flame exercise, as you breathe in to blow the candle flame, the diaphragm drops slightly. By placing your finger at the base of the sternum (breast-bone), where your lower ribs swing out to the side, you will feel the diaphragm thinning out at the mid-point where the ribs join in front, and pressing on your abdomen, and – if your baby is sufficiently high – also on the place where your baby's buttocks are. You feel the pressure inside and slightly towards the back; as you continue to breathe in, the sensation spreads out sideways towards your ribs.

Exercise 5

In the same way, if you take a deep breath, the diaphragm thins out and presses down as you do so. Then suddenly shout: 'Oh!'; you will feel it spring back into position very rapidly.

Types of Breathing

It is easy to be too dogmatic about what breathing to use when, and only a woman in labour can know what helps her most. But a general rule is that you think of your breathing as a bubble on the wave of the contraction. Each time the breathing is *on top* of the contraction. As contractions get bigger the breathing moves higher.

Practise these exercises lying on the floor rather than on a soft bed, and find a comfortable position; for instance, completely relaxed in the front lateral position, i.e. three-quarters over, with your head turned to one side, knees and elbows well flexed, and cushions wherever you want them (probably under your head and by the breasts). Allow yourself plenty of space so that you do not lie in a cramped position. An alternative position which many women prefer is to lie on the back, knees drawn up and apart, and cushions under the head and knees.

Exercise 1

Deep thoracic breathing (slow, full chest breathing). This is used as soon as contractions make the abdominal wall rigid, when you feel that you need to do something about meeting them. To practise, rest your hands at the sides of the ribs, spreading your fingers out so that you can feel as much of the bony cage as possible. Fill your lungs with air right down to the bottom, and you will feel your ribs swing out and up with each breath in, and swing down again with each breath out. These contractions last between thirty and fifty seconds, and the cervix is usually three to four centimetres dilated. The interval between contractions is anything from about seven to about ten minutes. Once you have mastered this type of breathing you will not need to have your hands on the ribs. Relax them by your sides.

Exercise 2

Upper thoracic breathing (quicker, shallow chest breathing). Now practise doing this more rapidly, when it is easier to use only the upper part of your chest, and you may like to breathe through your mouth to get the air more quickly. As the contractions get more powerful you may find this more comfortable, as it will leave the lower part of the body to get on with the work of pulling open the cervix. In practice, you do not need to adapt immediately by going straight into this shallow breathing for every contraction. Begin by taking a few deep, slow breaths and as the contraction mounts to its height the breathing becomes more rapid and lighter. It then slows down again and gets deeper as the contraction fades. The height of a contraction is approximately two-thirds of the way through, and it is then that you can breathe more quickly and lightly. Finish each contraction with a long breath out, and rest. These contractions last about one minute and the cervix is usually four or five centimetres dilated, or a little more. The interval between contractions is anything from about three and a half to about seven minutes.

Exercise 3

Mouth-centred breathing. If you breathe heavily and fast you are likely to hyperventilate. Symptoms are pins and needles in your hands and dizziness. So avoid this and, if you want to breathe more quickly to handle contractions, breathe more lightly. This light breathing can be used at the end of the first stage if you like, and is the shallowest and quickest type of breathing that you may want to do. To practise, relax the shoulders and neck muscles, drop the jaw and breathe in and out through the mouth. Start slowly at first or you may find yourself gasping. It should be rhythmic and easy. Concentrate on sensations in the mouth rather than in the throat, or you may feel the air is 'catching' in the throat and you may cough. Your head should be inclined slightly forward and your body relaxed. You may notice that your whole body seems to shake slightly; it is bound to do so if you are relaxed.

If you find this hard – and it is one of the more difficult kinds of breathing to learn – think of an old-fashioned steam train in the distance; start very slowly and speed up as you get the knack of it.

Your partner's help with this is useful. He can press your leg to simulate a uterine contraction, timing it with a watch. He increases pressure up to the crest of each one, two-thirds of the way through. Late first-stage contractions last about one minute, and the interval between them is usually anything from one minute to about three minutes. Start the contraction slowly by breathing in and out deeply; then in again; drop the jaw and commence with the shallow chest breathing as you 'feel' for the rhythm of the contraction. As it begins to mount to its climax, centre the breathing in your mouth, till you reach the crest of the wave. Then the breathing begins to drop down, becoming slower and softer, till at the end of the contraction it fades away. Breathe out through your mouth, letting out as much stale air for as long as you can. Do not forget this, or you may lack oxygen when doing shallow breathing.

It is as well to rehearse this often, as shallow quicker breathing may be helpful at the most difficult stage of labour when contractions are strong and there is a very short interval between them.

Remember that your body stays relaxed and at peace. If your breathing becomes uneven you may get very tired, and this will mean not only that you are not on top of your form for the active second stage, but that you will feel pain much more readily.

A word of caution is necessary here. The pace and depth of the breathing is a matter of very subtle adjustment according to the intensity and duration of the contractions. Only the woman in labour herself can judge the exact speed of respiration which helps her at that time. Some women tend to 'over-breathe' – tackling the whole process so energetically and enthusiastically that they breathe at once too deeply and too quickly, and this may result in excessive loss of carbon dioxide from the lungs. A certain amount of carbon dioxide is usually residual in the lungs and acts as the normal stimulus to respiration. When this is flushed out giddiness, pins and needles in the fingers and even cramp result. If you notice these signs your breathing should be more relaxed and less vigorous. It is important both in pregnancy and labour that you should experiment to find the right breathing *for you*.

Mouth-centred breathing is also used through the transition phase between the first and second stages of labour, when it occurs (some women go straight from the first to the second stage). Contractions during transition often become very irregular in type, duration and in the interval between them, and you may be starting to get the urge to push during this phase. Shallow, rapid breathing is also used when the baby's head crowns.

There may be a phase after you are fully dilated and before you have a passionate urge to push, however, when the uterus has pressed the baby's head through the cervix and contractions continue, but are much less strong. Sometimes you can hardly feel them at all. They may get farther apart, too. This lasts a few minutes, or two or three hours. *It does not mean that your uterus has stopped working and that you have gone out of labour.* When this happens, you are able to breathe more fully and slowly again. Do not exhaust yourself by pushing just because your cervix is fully dilated. This is what I call a 'rest and be thankful' transition. There is a hill outside Edinburgh at the top of which is a bench on which to rest and look down on the city. Inscribed on it are the words, 'Rest and be thankful'. You are within sight of your baby's birth, so use this time to relax completely and gain strength for the active second stage.

Exercise 4

Diaphragmatic breathing.[7] This is used for the expulsion of the baby in the second stage. To practise, breathe in, blow out; then take a deep breath in through the mouth, fixing the ribs and diaphragm, and, holding your breath, with your chin tucked in against your chest, and arms relaxed by your side and slightly flexed at the elbows, lean on the cushion of intra-abdominal

---

[7] All breathing necessarily involves the diaphragm, but in this type the diaphragm is used for pressing the baby down.

pressure you can feel beneath the diaphragm and press down firmly and slightly outwards, feeling the muscles which will help you to squeeze your baby gently and evenly down the birth canal, deliberately *releasing the muscles of the pelvic floor.* It may help to think of a tube of toothpaste which you are rolling up from the end with steady pressure. Avoid all erratic straining and check that you are using only those muscles which are necessary to the action. In this type of breathing all pressure is from *above*, your diaphragmatic muscles helping the contracting uterus to press the baby down. There is no need to pull with your hands; that is a waste of muscular effort and will tend to make you tighten up. Nor is there need to pull the abdominal muscles in to perform this action; they should be released. You will feel the pressure pass right down through the abdomen until it is on the pelvic floor and you feel your vulva open wide.

In labour, if the contraction is still powerful and you have finished pushing, you will want to take some more breaths quickly and press down again. But only push when and for as long as you feel the urgent desire to do so. When you are actually giving birth you won't have to think about how you are breathing, any more than you would think how you are breathing when you experience orgasm. You will find yourself breathing quickly as you become more excited and then your breath is held involuntarily. Contractions of the expulsive type last between thirty and forty seconds and the interval between them is anything from half a minute to about two minutes. As the baby gets lower the contractions may change their nature and you get a succession of weak ones following some very powerful ones. It is important to adapt yourself to this and press down only as firmly as the contractions indicate. You may also notice that you get an occasional longer interval for rest between contractions, and should take full advantage of this to relax completely and breathe deeply.

It is a good idea to rehearse this kind of breathing occasionally when practising relaxation, or try to get to bed a little earlier and imagine yourself giving birth before you go to sleep. You can rehearse pressing the baby down when you are on the lavatory, too. It is an effective remedy for constipation.

It is important to emphasise again that only you can tell when it is best to use each type of breathing. If contractions start coming at intervals of less than seven minutes and are powerful you may find you handle them best with mouth-centred breathing immediately labour begins. This may happen if your labour is induced. It can also occur after artificial rupture of the membranes. If you have a fast labour rapid adjustment is necessary, and quick evaluation of the contractions and the right breathing response to them. On the other hand, you may be happy breathing slowly and fully through even huge contractions.

Practising breathing with Braxton-Hicks contractions

Contractions of the uterus occur not only in labour but throughout pregnancy. Before labour starts the 'trial' contractions are known as Braxton-Hicks contractions. You are unlikely to notice these until the later months of pregnancy. First, you may think that it is the baby moving, but you will notice that if you lay a hand on your abdomen it is hard, protuberant and firm, and that as the movement dies down the abdominal wall becomes relatively soft again. It feels a little as if the baby were turning a somersault, but at the point when it has half turned it stays rigid and immobile for some seconds. That is the height of the contraction, and sometimes it is so strong and feels so surprising that you find yourself holding your breath. Don't! Breathe through it instead. These contractions are of the same nature as those experienced in labour, but when labour starts they recur at regular intervals.

If you get the opportunity to relax while watching trees swaying in a storm, practise adapting yourself to a rhythm which is rather like that of labour. Lie or sit and check that you have complete muscular release. Keeping your eyes on the branches in the wind, feel your relaxed body adjust to the sweep of the storm, and you will discover that your breathing rhythm has altered and is following the movement of the biggest branches as they are driven in a wide arc by the wind. The branches do not crack because they go *with* the wind and do not resist it. They bend and give with the storm in much the same way as you will find harmony in your labour.

SECOND STAGE CO-ORDINATION

Pushing

It is commonly supposed that the abdominal muscles need to be used forcefully in expulsive effort during the second stage of labour. In childbirth classes women may be taught how to use these muscles and to press the abdominal wall in on to the contracting uterus. They are taught how to relax them for the first stage of labour, but are expected to be able to contract them for the second stage. This is not only unnecessary but undesirable. The action by which the baby is pressed down the birth canal should be piston-like, with all pressure exerted from above on to the fundus of the uterus, and the muscles of the perineum completely relaxed. If the abdominal wall is drawn taut and pressed in on the contracting uterus, pressure is exerted on the sides of the uterus and in this way the pressure from above is prevented from having its full effect.

If you hold a cardboard cylinder in your hand and press a marble through it from the top (with a finger of the other hand performing the role of the diaphragm) the journey will be made rather more difficult if you grip the cylinder firmly than if you release the pressure.

Think of your uterus as a large avocado pear or fig, the stalk of which lies below your diaphragm at the mid-point of your abdomen, and which is tilted down towards your buttocks. Take a deep breath in, fix your ribs and diaphragm and, holding your breath, feel as if you are pressing down from the stalk end right through the whole pear shape till you reach the very bottom of it. It will help to feel as if you are leaning on a bolster of air. If you place your cupped hands at the bottom of your abdomen, just where you begin to curve in again, you will feel your muscles pushing your hands down and out away from your body.[8] Press down from the diaphragm until you feel the movement on your pelvic floor and your vagina will automatically open up.

Now do the opposite movement, pressing your abdominal wall in hard. You will see that it is much more difficult to relax your vagina at the same time, and that the movement is rather uncomfortable, making you feel as if you are being laced into an old-fashioned corset. The baby will still be born if you do this, but the movement may constrict the contracting uterus. A woman who is unafraid and fully aware will spontaneously use the previous movement rather than this one, and will be right in her instinctive response to the message coming from her uterus.

To practise bearing down in this way, lie on a bed or couch well supported with pillows, with your partner sitting at your side with an arm around you. See that the lower part of your spine – the sacrum and coccyx – is lying flat on the surface of the bed. After you have practised the bearing down movement once or twice your partner can interrupt you and say 'Stop', and you instantly stop and start panting lightly so that the baby's head can be born more slowly as you 'breathe it out'. You may want to reach down and touch it.

Toning your Pelvic Floor and Relaxing your Vagina

It is important to know how to mobilise the muscles of the pelvic floor, how to release them while the baby is being born, and keep them firmly toned following the baby's birth. You can learn to isolate and control these muscles so that they can be released and contracted at will and their tone increased. This is one of the most important exercises a woman can do, whether pregnant or not.

---

[8] Some women find it easiest to think of a pyramid, the base of which is formed by the big hip-bones and the top of which is formed by the centre of the diaphragm. They exert pressure from that point right down through to the base at its widest.

Exercise 1

First, pull in all the muscles in and around your vagina, *without tensing your thighs or buttocks*. Pull them in, draw them up as strongly as you can, and hold. Then release them so that they are quite soft and seem to be falling away from you like a hammock from the large bones of your pelvis. As they are released it may help to think of a lift going right down to the bottom floor of a high building. Check that you release the muscles completely and do not stop three-quarters of the way down. Now release them that little bit more. Finally, pull in and hold.

Exercise 2

Draw in and tighten the very powerful sphincter of the anus (back passage) without tensing the muscles around your vagina directly. Do this very gently and slowly, or you will find that the movement passes through into the vagina as well. Since the *levator ani*, although composed of different muscular segments, stretches right across the perineum, it is impossible to isolate each completely, but experiment to see how delicate a muscular control you can achieve. Then deliberately release the muscles. Finish by pulling in again.

Exercise 3

Now feel as if you are constricting a ring of muscle about half-way up inside your vagina, like a kiss inside, and at the same time draw up and in the muscles that are just underneath your pubis.[9] Most of the tightening should be at the front and you feel only a slight ripple of muscular contraction towards the anus. You will feel the ring tighten to an oval, getting narrower, till you can imagine holding a hazelnut in with these muscles. The top circle of what is like a figure eight of muscle tightens, while the transverse perineal muscle that stretches across where the two circles meet is drawn forward towards your pubis. Hold it, and then release the muscles. Finally, pull them in again.

---

[9] See diagram on p. 53.

Exercise 4

There is a still deeper level of muscle inside the front passage, nearer your bladder. Now pull in the ring of muscle you have just been exercising, and then draw up and in the muscles just underneath your pubis, at about the level of the hair line. If you rest your fingers there you will be able to feel the pull deep inside. These muscles help support your bladder. Then release them. Then pull them in again.

If you are uncertain of the effect you are creating as you concentrate on these muscular contractions, experiment in the bath and insert the tip of one finger, first in the anus and then in the vagina. In this way you will be able to judge the effectiveness and precision of what you are trying to do. Stream-stopping when you are passing urine will also help you to control and strengthen these muscles. After doing this always relax and finish emptying your bladder completely.

Exercise 5

Once you have achieved this delicate control, practise tightening the *glutei* (the buttock muscles), and then pulling in the muscles of the pelvic floor. Imagine that you have a sheet of paper between your buttocks and someone is trying to pull it out. Hold it for a moment and then release the *glutei while keeping the muscles of the pelvic floor firmly contracted*. Difficult, but it comes with practice. Now release these muscles too.

Exercise 6

Press the tops of your legs towards each other, tightening your adductors – the muscles of your inside thighs – without contracting your pelvic floor muscles. Then relax and let your legs flop apart. Now tighten the tops of your legs again and then pull in your pelvic floor. Still holding your adductors tight, relax your pelvic floor. Then relax completely.

You will see that you do not need to contract either buttock muscles or muscles in your legs to contract your pelvic floor. Pelvic floor exercises are invisible ones. And you can do them anywhere. Use times when you have to stand and wait to mobilise these muscles.

Exercise 7

There are muscles further at the back, just where your tail would be if you had one. Babies often have a deep dimple there. See if you can wag the tail up and down. Now relax. These muscles sometimes tighten when a woman in labour feels the bump of the baby's head coming down and pressing against her anus. She may worry that she wants to empty her bowels. If she is sitting on a bed she may lift her buttocks up off the bed. If you release these muscles you can help your baby's head down to be born.

This delicate muscular co-ordination does not come easily at first. When you have an internal examination during your pregnancy you can check with your doctor or midwife that you are doing this correctly. It is easy to feel when you are gripping the examining finger or when you are pushing it out, but you may need practice to achieve complete muscular release there.

As your baby's head is being born you will have to release all these muscles or you may be torn or have an episiotomy (a cut), and whilst you hardly feel that at the time, it can be uncomfortable afterwards for some weeks.

Each time you finish rehearsing these movements, particularly when you have been imagining helping the baby's head bulge forward, remember to contract the muscles smoothly and firmly so that you complete the exercise by toning them.

Association between Mouth and Vagina

When we want something too much and concentrate our thoughts on it to the exclusion of all else, the very opposite may result. This is particularly true with relaxation of any part of the body. When the baby's head, feeling very large indeed, is pressing solidly against the pelvic floor, it is easy to tense up those muscles even when you are trying to release them.

Muscular release can be greatly helped at this point by having trained yourself during the later months of pregnancy in conscious association between the part of the body which is under stress and another part which is not under stress.

There is an unconscious neuro-muscular association between the vagina and the mouth. The pads of flesh at either side of the vagina are even called labia (lips). Our earliest experiences of delight are centred in our mouths and lips, associated with pleasurable feeding. Even when our eroticism has developed to full genital maturity we retain pleasure in stimulation of the surfaces of the lips and tongue, which are still sensitive to touch: we enjoy kissing; some people smoke; others chew gum or sweets or chocolates. We never entirely outgrow our early mouth-centredness.

When a woman is tense in the region of the pelvic floor she can often be helped to relax by being shown how to relax her mouth and jaw. If I then ask her to get the same feeling of looseness in her vagina she can do it easily. If she starts tightening her mouth, she finds that she is automatically tightening up the pelvic floor, too.

In photographs of mothers giving birth without laceration they often have their mouths open as the baby's head is crowning and being born. They are smiling or laughing, lips parted in pleasure and excitement. In old-fashioned midwifery it was sometimes customary to instruct the mother to scream or shout as the baby's head started to bulge through the perineum. This must have afforded release of tension, since you cannot scream fully unless your jaw is dropped and mouth wide open.

Exercise 1

To build up an association between mouth and vagina, start by inclining your head forward and releasing the muscles of your lips, throat and tongue. Your jaw should feel as if it is hanging from your cheekbones and from just below your ears. If you put your fingertips over those points and then let your jaw drop, it may prove easier. Feel as if you are wearing very heavy earrings. See that the tip of your tongue is resting against the back of the lower front teeth and your lips are slightly parted. At the same time feel the soft palate spread wider apart and relaxed, opening out from the shape of a Gothic to a Roman arch. Now

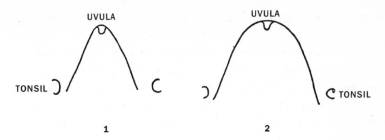

Diagrammatic representation of the movement of the soft palate as its muscles are released.
1. Here the palato-pharyngeal arch is contracted. This sort of contraction results when you feel as if a pill is stuck in your throat.
2. Here the palato-pharyngeal arch is relaxed.

concentrate on your vagina and tense up all those muscles hard. Involuntarily, you will discover, you have tightened muscles in your throat, your jaw has become rigid, and that you have either curled the tip of your tongue back or started to push it against your front teeth.

Exercise 2

Now release the muscles of your mouth and pelvic floor and start again, but this time relax your pelvic floor first. Then relax your mouth. Now firmly clench your teeth, tighten your lips, throat and tongue. If the birth outlet is still relaxed you have quite extraordinary control. Now relax both mouth and pelvic floor. Keep them relaxed like this for a minute or so. Breathe in and out gently and slowly through your parted lips, and at the same time feel as if you are breathing with your vagina.

This is what you want your body to do when the baby's head is being pressed through the outlet. Imagine that you have the baby's head much the size of a grapefruit in your vulva, and help it bulge forward by releasing the muscles in this way. Every time you rehearse pushing, especially when rehearsing the panting breathing you can use when the head crowns and when you want to stop pushing, *relax your mouth* and let your jaw drop from your cheekbones. Be particularly careful that when you pant you do not at the same time tense up your lips and throat. Your head should be well tilted forward on to your chest.

When you are in labour and your baby is about to make an entry into the world it is extremely difficult to know yourself whether you are relaxing your vagina. The feeling of the baby's head is so unfamiliar that it hardly seems like the body you know any more. It is like a seed pod bursting open, or like the speeded-up films of flowers opening in sunlight in TV natural history programmes. But you can tell what you are doing with your mouth. So as the baby approaches the perineum, gradually fans it out and then slowly oozes through the vagina, concentrate on releasing your lips, tongue and throat, and it will be much easier.

'In normal labour . . . during the second stage, the uterine contractions exert a force proportional to the resistance of the lower genital canal; the perineum is able to bear all the force instinctively exerted without injury,' as Thomas Denman wrote over a hundred years ago,[10] but if the woman, from excitement or from pain, begins to use all her force to end the labour speedily we know that there is a grave risk of laceration of the perineum.

---

[10] Thomas Denman, *An Introduction to the Practice of Midwifery*, 6th edn, London, 1829.

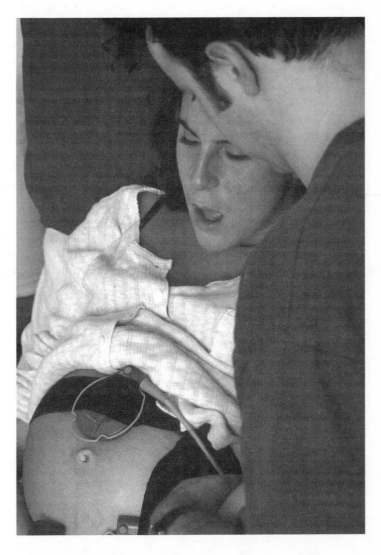

Having a birth companion on whom you can rely
utterly frees you to concentrate on the power released
in your body and to work with it.

6

A Note to Partners

'I thought the best husbands looked on their wives' lying in as a
time of festival and jollity. What? Did you not even get drunk in
the time of your wife's delivery? Tell me honestly how you employed yourself at this time.'

'Why then honestly,' replied he, 'and in defiance of your
laughter, I lay behind her bolster and supported her in my arms.'

Henry Fielding, *Amelia*, first published in 1751

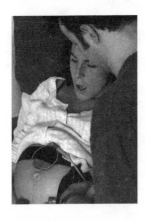

Throughout this book I refer to the
presence of the father, and it is against
him that a woman may lean as she
gives birth to the child. Perhaps he is
the first person to see the baby and it
may even be in his arms that it first falls
asleep.

This is the right place for a father to
be. It is not only ludicrous but pathetic
to leave him to stride up and down
a hospital corridor, while the woman
'gets on with it' alone.

'The last requirement of all for a successful delivery at home
is the husband – the poor father. If he is of the right mentality,
and very few are, he may sustain his wife's morale during the
first part of her labour. Otherwise he is best employed making
tea, keeping the kettles boiling, and answering the front door
bell.' Thus was the father condescendingly referred to in a
rather dated BMA publication, *You and Your Baby*. We are not
told how many pots of tea and how many kettles of water
he succeeded in boiling at the end of a sixteen-hour labour,
nor what anyone was going to do with it all. As occupational
therapy it is perhaps as good as anything, but it is wasteful, and

denies the woman in labour the reassurance, active assistance and loving care of the father of this child who is making its way into the world.

There is no need for the father to be the figure of fun that he is in so many TV sitcoms, treated as if he had neither the intelligence nor the humanity to be of any help.

On the other hand, a partner – whether male or female – who is present without having a clue as to how to help may not only feel superfluous but be in the way. I have written as if a partner is always male, but a woman partner brings with her to birth her own experiences, too. Has she wanted a baby but been unable to have one? Has she had a miscarriage? Is she anxious or frightened about birth? Or has she had a positive birth experience herself? A partner who understands labour as a process of which the birth is the natural climax – not an isolated, traumatic and shocking occurrence – is extremely unlikely to faint, in spite of all the apocryphal stories about fathers passing clean out on the floor that are part of midwifery tradition. As one new father put it, 'I could never bear having an injection or the sight of blood. I'm squeamish about these things generally, but when you are there from the beginning and have a job to do – rubbing her back and helping her with her breathing – then there is no shock involved. It all seems perfectly natural.'

To be most helpful I suggest that a partner does the following:

During Pregnancy

Read some of the books on childbirth she is reading. Discuss them with her.

Go with her at least once when she visits her midwife to discuss her birth plan.

Help with her exercises.

Let her see that he has complete confidence in her and in her capacity to have her baby naturally.

Learn from other fathers' experiences. Visit www.Fathers Direct.com

During Labour

If the birth is to be at home, prepare the room. The best lighting is indirect lighting or candlelight with a side light from a standard or table lamp. Pull the bed out at right angles to the wall if it is not already in this position and help make it up with old sheets and a waterproof sheet underneath. (Many women like a painting or a bowl of flowers to concentrate on during contractions.)

Stay with her throughout labour if that is what she wants.

Be calm.

Explain to the midwife or obstetrician what she is trying to do if they do not understand. Insist that she is given no analgesia unless she agrees to it. A birth companion's task is not, of course, to *prevent* her accepting analgesics, but rather to see that they are not – as occasionally happens – forced upon her if she feels she does not require them.

Be ready with early contractions to massage her back firmly in the sacral area – near where the big hip-bones join the spine, or massage her hips and thighs if she has pain there.

Refresh and stimulate her with sips of raspberry leaf tea, fruit juice, water, strong, sweet black coffee or other drinks if she wants them.

As the end of the first stage approaches, wring out sponges or face cloths in very cold, preferably iced, water, and rest them against her forehead, the nape of her neck, and possibly also over her lips. An electric fan also may help if she is feeling very hot.

Give her an extra duvet and hot water bottles if she feels shivery at the end of the first stage. She will probably appreciate a hot water bottle at her feet, and one tucked in the small of her back may help to relieve pain.

Give her barley sugar, or sugar, or anything sweet to suck if she wants it. This helps her keep up her energy.

Help her into an upright or all fours position for the second stage, and give physical support if she needs it.

Do not take over. The woman giving birth leads. You follow. If she wants to make a noise – fine!

IN HOSPITAL

It can be one thing learning how to rub a woman's back or hold her so that she can bear down effectively in the friendly atmosphere of a small antenatal class where couples are working together, often with much discussion interspersed with laughter, and quite another to carry the same confidence into a large, perhaps rather impersonal, hospital where you are confronted in labour with professionals in white or green whom you have never met before, whose names you do not know, in a strange, clinical environment where, in spite of consent by the hospital to your presence, you feel out of place. Both parents-to-be may feel that they are entering alien and even 'enemy' territory and that nobody will understand or sympathise with what they are trying to do.

For having a baby in a big hospital means that the couple have to enter a bureaucratic system. Authority is organised in a pyramidal structure, with the patients at the bottom of it, and power over other people is distributed and legitimised by administrative machinery which, because its main aims are economy and efficiency, can often make care impersonal.

Some hospitals are also frustrating places for those working in them. Hospital midwives have to act dual roles and so are often in a difficult position themselves. They are directly responsible for the care of their patients, but also have to execute administrators' and obstetricians' decisions. The odd thing about nursing and midwifery is that the staff who have most direct contact with patients have lowest status, and those farthest removed from the patient have highest status. As midwives move up in their profession they tend to go into administrative, office-based jobs. This means that the most experienced midwives have little or no contact with patients. Maternity patients often find that they achieve most personal contact with student midwives, for example, or even the 'tea lady', and in teaching hospitals they may find the medical student told to sit in on the labour a great deal more approachable than the senior consultant.

In one study of 'problem patients' it was found that those

presenting no difficulty from nurses' point of view were those who complied with instructions willingly, made no demands and asked no questions, so that nurses could get on with their work. 'Problem patients', on the other hand, slowed down the nurses' work, interrupted the smooth flow of activity and asked too many questions.

It helps if the couple going into hospital are aware of some of the organisational problems with which staff have to cope and realise that there are stresses and strains in the lives of midwives and doctors, too. It is also important for them to become familiar with this alien environment in order to be able to function effectively in it and make positive relationships with members of staff.

A couple going into hospital and asking to be kept fully informed of what is happening, and to share in the decision-making about the labour, are pioneering for other parents who come after them who, perhaps, may find it more difficult to express themselves and ask for what they want. Each woman having a baby acts not only for herself, but for all those others who also have a right to be treated not only as patients, but as people, and not as reproductive machines but as individuals.

Yet doctors and midwives are people too! It can do nothing but harm to go into hospital with banners flying, incense burning, and a list of commands, aggressively confronting members of staff as the combined opposition!

The key to achieving good communication and explaining what you would like is to get a note down on your records in advance, to the effect that you would like your labour to be as natural as possible. It is also important to know and, if possible, address people by name. If for example the woman in labour likes her legs stroked, her partner sitting on the bed with his arms round her, or a hot water bottle in the small of her back, or to squat instead of lying in bed, she should not say: 'That's what I learned to do in classes' as if it were a set of rules which she is presenting but rather, 'I find this very helpful.' With this kind of approach, many couples are pleasantly surprised at how delighted midwives are to work along with them.

In more and more hospitals midwives and doctors welcome

patients who have learned how to help themselves and have some understanding of the processes of childbirth. I was in one large teaching hospital with a woman in labour and thanked the midwife for letting me be there. She said, 'Oh, it is lovely having a mother with a natural birth! We do appreciate it!' Later she watched the woman as she peacefully breathed her way through a contraction, an expression of almost sensuous satisfaction on her face, and said, 'It looks really, well, pleasurable, having a baby!' Each woman who gives birth with joy influences the midwives and doctors who attend her and makes it more possible for other women to have a similar experience.

How the Birth Partner can Help with a Technologically Controlled Labour

It is a good idea for the man as well as the woman to see round the maternity unit before the baby is due; most hospitals now have a system whereby small groups can see the labour and delivery suite.

When couples are there they should ask to see any apparatus that might be used in labour, such as the oxytocin drip which stimulates contractions to induce or accelerate labour, and the monitoring equipment which records the pressure of contractions and the baby's heartbeat. Women sometimes say that it was when they were approached with this equipment, which was unfamiliar and frightening, that they began to tense up, and that if they had known what it looked like before, and how it worked, they would have found it much easier to stay relaxed, and would have thought through whether or not they were willing to give their consent to its use.

Men who have been giving good support to their partners before equipment of this kind is used sometimes give up when they feel that the machinery has 'taken over'. This is understandable, because when a drip stand or monitoring equipment is beside the bed it is physically more difficult to get close to the woman, and when an external monitoring belt, which fits round her abdomen, is used it is difficult to massage the bottom of the bulge.

In most hospitals, if the labour is monitored and speeded up, the intimacy that the couple may have had together in earlier labour is lost, and this can lead to a feeling that the experts with their machinery have completely taken over. But there is no reason why emotional support and loving care should be withdrawn because modern technology is being used. The right place for the man is still at the woman's side, at the head end of the bed. There may not be room for a chair when the equipment is trundled in, but there is nearly always space for a stool, or he can just stand.

If he can no longer stroke his partner's tummy, there are other kinds of touch which can help her. It is often useful to hold her shoulder firmly during big contractions, and if she has previously practised relaxing so that she 'flows out towards' his touch, this will help her to keep her shoulders loose, and avoid over-breathing. Between contractions they can talk about where she likes to be stroked or held.

Since lying flat on her back may result in postural hypotension, and because the uterus presses on large blood vessels, reducing blood flow to the placenta, it is not a good position for labour. If she is lying down the blood flow through the placenta to the baby is at its fullest when she is on her side. This is why she may be asked to lie on her left side if monitoring equipment is used, or during a long labour. It is not a good idea for her to lie still for long periods, and she can ask her partner to help her roll over on to the other side occasionally. If she has an external monitor, the 'corset' will probably need adjusting then. It may be necessary to check that the clip has not come off the baby's head if the monitoring device has been introduced through her cervix. If she is sitting up, supported by four or five pillows, or is in any other upright posture, there is not the same problem of decreased blood flow to the baby.

An oxytocin drip aims at stimulating the uterus into activity as similar to that of normal labour as possible. But it often produces contractions which are extremely powerful from the start and come about every two minutes. This means that the breathing techniques to handle contractions of this magnitude may need to be those of the late first stage, even though she is only just starting to dilate.

One problem with modern equipment is that men often get fascinated by it, and may get so involved with watching the monitor, for example, that the woman takes second place, and feels that love and emotional support have been withdrawn from her. The man should not forget that, however sophisticated the machinery, it is she who is having the baby. Once labour is well under way, *his attention should be on her, and encouragement by word, touch or look, be given with every single contraction.*

Another problem may be that from the hospital's side, too, an induced or speeded-up and monitored labour becomes an interesting clinical exercise. Students may come in to watch. Teaching may go on at the bedside. Discussions about the equipment sometimes take place while the woman is busy with a contraction and would appreciate silence so that she could concentrate better. Although you cannot ensure that everyone is quiet during contractions, you can indicate politely by your silence and attention to her that you are not available for conversation during contractions, and by doing this can help her enter a 'circle of solitude' with you and the baby who is coming to birth.

AFTER THE BIRTH

Birth is only the beginning. Once the child is born a woman should feel that however bad a mother she thinks she is, however she fails, however others criticise her, *her partner* believes in her.

Her partner should also be quick to see how and when to help. They may be able to learn something from each other in their handling of the baby. When parenthood is a shared enterprise it is more fun for both.

Childbirth is not an illness, but work for which the female body is efficiently and most exquisitely constructed. It should take place in an atmosphere of tranquillity and loving care.

Teams of skilled staff, batteries of sterile instruments, rows of antiseptically clean and shining delivery rooms, and spotless nurseries shielded by plate glass cannot achieve this. But the comfort of home, the friendly care of a midwife and the support of a partner who cherishes the woman and shares with her pleasure in the baby's birth – these in themselves take a woman a long way towards childbirth which brings with it exultant joy.

And the purpose of it all – the baby. A new father greets his child:

> 'As for the baby, I was frightened by it. Such frailty; the paper-thin, yet powerful, cry. A living being, warm and wet from the womb, utterly helpless, bemused, staring about with bright eyes. Tiny fingers and fingernails plucking at the air. Perhaps it is a sense of responsibility that frightens me, or some primeval feeling of guilt. I have helped to create a life; a pulsing being that might be crushed sooner or later in a million different ways; a small accident, an illness, in a cataclysm. Yet the baby having been born, one feels its journey is ended, not just begun. That it should suffer the risks of life seems unfair. Before this tiny presence those risks seem formidable. One is acutely aware of the preciousness of life. One drives with extra care this day. One sees people about one as more real people.'[1]

Laurie Lee, in 'The Firstborn',[2] is stirred by the same helplessness:

> She was born in the autumn and was a late fall in my life, and lay purple and dented like a little bruised plum, as though she'd been lightly trodden in the grass and forgotten.
>
> Then the nurse lifted her up and she came suddenly alive, her bent legs kicking crabwise, and her first living gesture was a thin wringing of the hands accompanied by a far-out Hebridean lament.

---

[1] See Sheila Kitzinger, *Giving Birth: Emotions in Childbirth*, Sphere, 1979.
[2] *I Can't Stay Long*, Penguin Books, 1981.

This moment of meeting seemed to be a birthtime for both of us; her first and my second life. Nothing, I knew, would be the same again, and I think I was reasonably shaken. I peered intently at her, looking for familiar signs, but she was convulsed as an Aztec idol. Was this really my daughter, this purple concentration of anguish, this blind and protesting dwarf?

Then they handed her to me, stiff and howling, and I held her for the first time and kissed her, and she went still and quiet as though by instinctive guile, and I was utterly enslaved by her flattery of my powers.

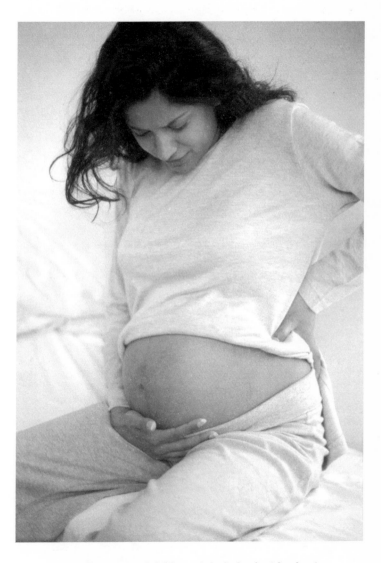

Contractions are felt like a tight belt of wide elastic
pulling in where your cervix is opening, and often in
the small of your back, too.

7
The Beginnings of Labour

He cam al so stylle,
There his moder was,
As dew in Aprille
That fallyt on the gras.
He came al so stylle
To his moderes bour,
As dew in Aprille
That fallyt on the flour.
He came al so stylle
There his moder lay,
As dew in Aprille
That fallyt on the spray.
Anonymous early fifteenth century.
(Quoted in *Broadway Book of English Verse*,
ed. W. B. Honey, Routledge, 1940)

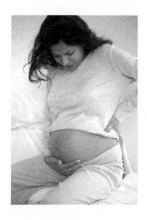

In birth a woman gives herself to the creative process and the transmission of life. It is not sufficient that she should have a baby inside her which is ripe to be born; she should long to savour the experience of birth to the full, and to express her joy in the birth through her body.

THE WOMAN'S ATTITUDE TO LABOUR

We approach birth with all sorts of preconceived ideas about what it will feel like, with hopes and fears of which we may not even be fully aware. Cultural factors influence a woman's acceptance of birth. Grantly Dick-Read drew attention to culturally induced fear of childbirth in our own society, in which stories relating to pain and endurance are handed down from mother to daughter and from older married women to young girls, stories which find a place in our literature and films and on TV. This culturally induced fear ranges through the whole gamut of literary and media output from light suggestion, epitomised by the heroine of the magazine romance whose labour pains are hinted at rather than described − ' "I must relax, I *must* relax," she muttered fiercely' − to the full realistic treatment of some TV sitcoms and films (though none the less often inaccurate). In the vivid scene − which I remember from my own childhood − in the film *Gone with the Wind* a woman is shown with the sweat streaming down her face during an agonising labour in which she later dies. The French film *Le Lit* showed a mother wincing with pain as the umbilical cord was cut! Nicolaiev in Russia and Lamaze in France based their teaching on destroying the unpleasant associations conditioned by society and re-educating the sympathetic nervous system. This is no simple task, for the cultural factors which they sought to neutralise also include the taboos which surround childbirth, the social sanctions which maintain and reinforce tradition, and the power of professionals in the medical system. Childbirth today is treated as a potentially pathological condition that needs to be managed in an intensive care setting.

Childbirth with joy is as much a matter of the mind as of the body and is as great an emotional as it is a physiological process.

A woman who is resisting and fighting her body can never enjoy the tussle of labour. She lies in stoic endurance, taut with anxiety, determined not to give in, or chooses to obliterate the sensations of birth with drugs. She retreats from the overwhelming reality of the childbirth experience.

Some women state their intention of having an epidural as early as possible in labour, or booking an elective Caesarean section to avoid the pain of labour. They usually know nothing about birth except that it hurts. Some of these women have suffered previous sexual abuse. For them it can be one way in which they feel able to take control.

In a normal, straightforward labour a woman's attitude of

mind is more important than any sort of physical preparation she can make in advance. Whatever athletic exercises she may practise, however controlled her breathing and complete her relaxation, in the last resort the thing that matters most is the person she is and the quality of the relationships with those who are caring for her. That is why *preparation for labour cannot rest in physical training and techniques of control.* Her ability to make the birth into something she creates rather than something she passively endures depends on her fearlessness, her sense of security because she is in a loving environment where she feels safe – and this includes not feeling that she is in a competition and has to prove herself a star performer – her joy in the baby's coming, courage, self-confidence, and the understanding she has of herself. *The experience she has of childbirth is a function of her whole personality* and ideally preparation for it should involve increased self-knowledge and a growing towards maturity.

To a woman who is looking to her partner for help and loving understanding of her fears and hopes, his psychological withdrawal is not only disappointing, but may be a severe shock at a critical phase in their relationship. She cannot help comparing him with other men who welcome the birth of their child as an experience to be shared. Occasionally a man who is very unwilling to be present will consent to be there if his partner insists. Each woman must judge for herself the wisdom of this, but on the whole anyone who dreads being at the birth is best left out of the reckoning.

There is another type of man who half-heartedly agrees to be at the birth if his partner really wants it but who refuses to read a book on the subject or help her with exercises – who thinks, perhaps, that he is too 'manly' for this, or who finds it all too painfully embarrassing. He may simply not have the imagination to understand her need of him.

A man who is not well-informed and has yet agreed to be at the birth is unlikely to know what he can do to help her and even a perfectly straightforward labour may be distressing for him. He does not understand what she is doing and feels completely out of place, and even though he is in the same room, she must feel a barrier of non-understanding.

Sometimes when a woman has a private obstetrician she fixes her affection on the doctor as a parent figure who must care for her and let her come to no harm – who will be firm, kind and loving. Research in different countries shows that a woman who has a private obstetrician is much more likely to have a Caesarean section or a delivery assisted by forceps or ventouse (a vacuum extractor), if only because obstetricians tend to see all birth in terms of pathology and are not experts in normal birth.

Many women need a woman with them who is like a mother. The midwife may fill this role well, especially if she is an older woman – and some women prefer more mature midwives, and worry in advance that a younger substitute will turn up when they are in labour. Even a sophisticated woman may suddenly feel this need for an older woman whom she can trust. It is important that she should have known the midwife long enough to have built up a relationship with her, and the midwife should stay with her from the onset of difficult contractions, and not leave her, or introduce a substitute.

But not all women want this, and resent an over-motherly midwife who laps 'her' patient in endearments and solicitude, cosseting her with a kindness which some more independent women find intensely irritating and irrelevant. Indeed, occasionally a (usually older) midwife will use her kindness to get power over her patient and, behind the 'lassies', 'dearies' and 'pets', one feels there lies a will of iron that must not be thwarted. I have seen a determined midwife try to force gas-and-oxygen on a woman in labour who was meeting difficulty during the last few contractions of the first stage, but who insisted that she did not want the mask. The midwife was deeply concerned at what seemed to her the stoic attitude of her patient. She said, 'You *must* have it, dear. I can't bear to see anyone in pain.' Struggling to get away from her, the woman replied, 'But I'm not in pain. I'm having contractions.' 'Well,' the midwife asserted, 'I can't bear to see anyone having contractions!' Then in desperation she exclaimed: 'Our Queen used it' – to which the woman answered, laughing even at the height of a big, late first-stage contraction, 'That doesn't cut any ice with me, Nurse. I'm an American.'

A midwife who finds her fulfilment in succouring helpless and frightened patients must find it richly rewarding when a woman is prepared to be completely dependent on her, but it is bound to lead to conflict when the woman has a mind of her own, and different ideas from those of the midwife.

When a woman and her midwife are in conflict with each other even a straightforward birth can be a traumatic experience. Midwives have a unique role, and the power to make this major life event satisfying or horrendous. They should never use this power to dominate and take over. There is an art in enabling a woman to find the way through birth that is right for her. It entails great sensitivity and skill, as well as being up-to-date with the research evidence that she needs to bear in mind. No woman should be coerced into having drugs for pain relief, or be refused medication when she wants it.

Being 'Overdue'

Babies are sometimes born exactly 280 days after the first day of the last period, but many are born as much as a fortnight later and sometimes they are earlier. Only about 5 per cent of women have their babies on the day they were expected, and the majority are about a week 'late'. First babies are very often late. Even using ultrasound dating methods, a baby may be born two weeks before the date you have been given or two weeks after, and still be on time. So it may be best not to give friends a precise due date. Otherwise they will be ringing up to say, 'Haven't you had it *yet?*' and you will be left feeling that you can't deliver the goods.

Some women agitate for labour to be induced if they think they are late, and some hospitals routinely induce if the baby is as much as a week 'overdue'. This is particularly fashionable in the USA. Induction involves drugs to stimulate the uterus into action, often together with puncturing and rupturing of the membranes if they have not already ruptured spontaneously. It is impossible to tell in advance how a uterus will respond to artificial stimulation. One serious disadvantage of induction with drugs to kick-start the uterus is that the labour may be characterised by irregular contractions varying in strength, some very strong ones being followed by others very weak, and the whole process be long drawn out or, especially if prostaglandins are used that are often employed for terminations, labour may be fast, furious and painful. This can be extremely tiring, and it is hard to adapt to a labour in which you are either having contractions the intensity of each of which you cannot foresee and when the interval between them is constantly altering, or one in which the uterus is hyper-stimulated, contractions are hard, long and almost non-stop, and there is risk of uterine rupture. Sometimes induction is advised for medical reasons because of pre-eclampsia or because the pregnancy is at forty-two weeks. There is evidence that, on average, babies do best if labour is induced then, rather than waiting longer.

But occasionally when labour has been induced for 'prolonged pregnancy' it is discovered that the baby was not, after all, overdue. The child born before it is ready for life is at a grave disadvantage. Induction should be avoided unless there are clear indications for it.

On the other hand, it must be remembered that the baby who is really overdue is also at a disadvantage. The placenta gradually becomes less efficient. Some of the signs that a baby was overdue are a very wrinkled skin, long fingernails that need cutting immediately, and chalky white areas on the placenta. This baby may need the same degree of care as a premature baby.

If you are waiting for labour to start, one way of stimulating the cervix to soften, and of perhaps initiating contractions, is to have sex, lying on your back with your heels on your partner's shoulders, so that semen, which is rich in prostaglandins, is deposited in and around the cervix. Continue lying on your back, hips raised on a pillow, afterwards. Your partner stimulates your nipples and, while you drift off to sleep, continues to do so every ten minutes or so for several hours.

Get out and about in the weeks before labour starts. Don't sit brooding about the length of your pregnancy. However, it is also important to have sufficient sleep; so parties should not go on too late. (Boredom, worry, and overtiredness are great threats to peace of mind as you start out on the adventure of childbirth.)

Once labour starts your body and mind are flooded with energy and any weariness felt in the hours before disappears. Many women have started labour after a full day's work and yet have not been tired. A warm bath, with aromatherapy oils to help you relax, and some steady deep breathing will help refresh you.

LABOUR STARTS

Waves rise, each to its individual height in a seeming attitude of unrelenting competition, but only up to a certain point; and thus we know of the great repose of the sea to which they are all related, and to which they must all return in a rhythm which is marvellously beautiful.

In fact, these undulations and vibrations, these risings and fallings, are not due to the erratic contortions of disparate bodies, they are a rhythmic dance. Rhythm can never be born of the haphazard struggle of combat. Its underlying principle must be unity, not opposition.

Rabindranath Tagore, Sadhana, *The Realisation of Life*.
Realisation in Love.

The signs of the preliminary labour phase are well known: a 'show' of blood-stained mucus (the gelatinous plug from the mouth of the uterus); odd contractions which feel something like menstrual pain; painless rupture of the membranes, either slowly by leaking, or in a gush. Any or all of these mean that the baby will probably be born within the next few days. Do not allow them to become signals for alarm. They are merely a sign that labour will begin shortly. Regular, rhythmic contractions which dilate the cervix are the only true indication that labour is under way.

If your membranes rupture before labour starts (premature rupture of the membranes) it is probably best not to go to hospital. The risk of infection is increased in hospital, especially if you have vaginal examinations. But it is sensible to take your temperature every four hours or so. If there is an infection your temperature will go up. Then you should let the midwife know. Contractions usually start within 12 hours of spontaneous rupture of the membranes. You are more likely to start labour naturally if you stay in the comfortable, familiar surroundings of home.

It is unwise to go into hospital until labour is well established, because you may concentrate on the inner mechanisms of your body before thinking about them can do any good at all. If you get impatient, it will help you relax to have a warm bath.

Be actively occupied until you feel you need to give your full attention to contractions. As they come, pause in whatever you are doing and follow them with full chest breathing, rising to shallow chest breathing if you need to. If you are standing release all those muscles which are not necessary and feel yourself hanging from the hips. If you have already practised relaxing while standing up this will come easily. If you are sitting, release all those muscles you do not need to use and, leaning slightly forward with rounded shoulders, feel the lower part of your body heavy whilst you bring your breathing into time with the contractions.

The contractions come like waves, last between thirty and sixty seconds at first, and their crest is about two-thirds of the way through. You will probably find that the uncomfortable gripping sensation around your pelvis and any pain radiating in the lumbar area disappears completely once you start breathing rhythmically and your partner is beside you rubbing your back, or very lightly massaging your lower abdomen. Regular, rhythmic breathing will help you control yourself if you are very excited.

It is important to start relaxing *before* you feel your body dominating you and before you find it difficult to release your muscles during contractions. Never try to talk during a contraction. As the first sensations of the contraction come *greet it with your breathing*. Take a full, deep breath, feeling your ribs swing out, without tightening your shoulders or chest or screwing up your eyes. Let it go slowly. Rest on the slight pause that naturally follows. Take another – rest on it – and then let it go gently and easily.

With winter babies it is important not to get chilled during labour, as it is extremely difficult to relax when cold. Wear a dressing gown and socks or have a pair of warm slippers which you can easily slip on. Since you are likely to spend some time in the lavatory the heating should be on.

Women whose breasts feel heavy are usually more comfortable if they keep a well-fitting bra on throughout labour.

If labour starts when you are in bed you will probably be able to doze off and on for some time, but if contractions are sharp and wake you it is important to wake up completely by splashing your face with cold water, drinking some hot coffee or tea, doing your face and hair, and getting things ready, or drowsiness will make it difficult to control your breathing and relaxation.

These early contractions are sometimes more difficult than ones coming much later in the first stage, not because they have more force, but because you have not yet adjusted to them. One woman who had been to my classes reported that she found it hard to control early first-stage contractions as it was very early morning and she was dozing between them, but when she woke up properly and started coping with her labour they were easy to deal with and, because of this, late first-stage contractions did not appear to be so powerful as these early ones.

If you bathe in the sea when the water is cold, putting your legs in first up to the thighs, they soon begin to adapt themselves to the icy water and feel warm, but as you lower the rest of your body into the water you realise with a shock that it is icy cold. Whilst the legs have adapted themselves to the temperature, the upper half has not yet had time to do so. It is the same with labour. A woman needs time to adapt herself to it.

Your partner should watch for any signs of tension and if you are in bed be the first to notice if you start to grip it, twist the sheet with your fingers, screw up your face, curl your toes or stiffen your shoulders. Any contractions of muscles at this phase of labour are likely to be increased as labour advances and subsidiary tensions are built up in sympathy with the increasingly strongly contracting uterus. You cannot afford this dispersal of energy.

THE PRESENTATION OF THE BABY

The baby's skull is not hard bone all over. There are 'soft spots' or fontanelles – a diamond-shaped one at the front and another smaller one at the back of the head, with a narrow gap connecting the two. During the second stage of labour, the skull is moulded by overlapping of the bones at these cranial vault sutures. The larger one is called the *bregma* or anterior fontanelle, and forms a space between the frontal and parietal bones. The smaller one at the back is called the posterior fontanelle, and lies between the occipital and parietal bones. Gradually, in the months after the birth, these ossify until the skull is all hard bone.

These fontanelles can be felt through the dilating cervix during the first stage of labour and in the birth canal during the second stage, and reveal which way the baby's head is lying. The presenting part of the fetus is that part which can be felt through the cervix. Either the head, brow, face, or breech (buttocks) can present, the first being by far the most usual.

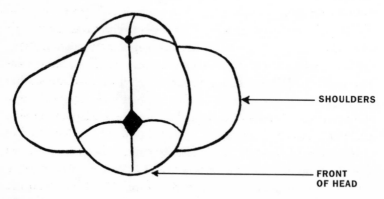

SHOULDERS

FRONT
OF HEAD

The baby's skull seen from above

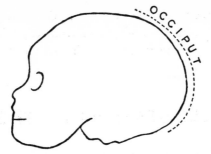

The baby's skull seen from the side

The More Usual Presentations

When labour begins the baby is usually in an anterior vertex position. That is, it is presenting by the head with the occiput towards the mother's front, either lying on the left or the right side. The obstetric terms for these are ROA (right occipito-anterior) and LOA (left occipito-anterior). The baby's head is usually well flexed forward on to its chest. The legs and arms are also flexed on to its body, and the baby is curled up like a hibernating dormouse.

Some Less Usual Presentations

Some babies lie in a posterior position, facing either right or left, and the occiput is then towards the mother's back. The obstetric terms for these are ROP (right occipito-posterior) and LOP (left occipito-posterior). This is a slightly less favourable position and often means a rather longer and more tedious labour, more severe backache, and greater strain on the maternal soft tissues. The mother with a baby in this position should not expect a rapid, easy labour. She needs to keep up her energy with sweetened drinks and sugar lumps or glucose, and possibly oxygen between contractions. The baby may be helped to flex itself further if she gets on all fours and rocks her pelvis, or she can lie on her left side when the occiput is on the right, and vice versa, using pillows and the weight of one leg to press on the baby to encourage its spine to flex. Or she can sit up with the

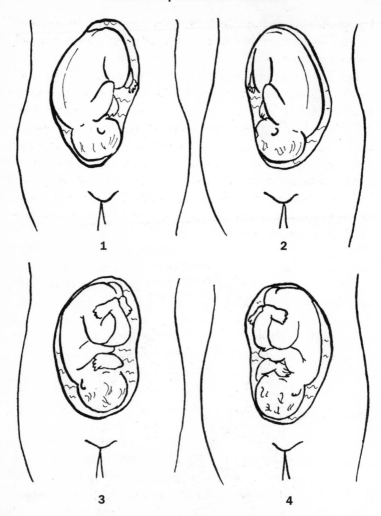

Some Positions the Baby may be in Before Labour Begins

Notice that these are all vertex presentations: i.e. the head is presenting.
1. Right occipito-anterior – ROA.
2. Left occipito-anterior – LOA – the most common position. In both ROA and LOA positions the baby is facing the mother's back. These are very good positions.
3. Right occipito-posterior – ROP.
4. Left occipito-posterior – LOP – a rare position. In both ROP and LOP positions the baby is facing the mother's front, and if the position persists (which it usually does not, since the baby rotates to an anterior position) it is born 'face to pubis'. These positions invariably mean a long first stage.

leg on the side against which the baby is lying raised on a stool or over the arm of the chair. In this position gravity will help rotation and descent.

A baby in a posterior position very often rotates into an anterior position at the very end of the first stage or during the second stage of labour, and you have to wait patiently while this takes place. Sometimes the baby begins to rotate but gets stuck in a transverse position (deep transverse arrest), and then help with forceps or a ventouse to suck the baby's head out is needed. This can happen when the mother has had an epidural which has removed the natural tone of the pelvic floor muscles. When the baby remains in a posterior position this is known as POP (persistent occipito-posterior).

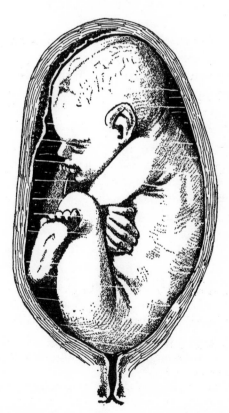

Breech Presentation

In face presentations the baby's head is not flexed on to its chest as it usually is, and unless the baby's head is small labour may be slower and some help may be needed with the birth. In brow presentations the brow is presenting; this is rare.

In breech births the first stage of labour is often slow, although after the baby is born to the buttocks it is important that its head should slip out fairly quickly, so the doctor or midwife usually does an episiotomy so that the head can be delivered more rapidly.

In breech deliveries a mother who is alert can help a great deal by bearing down when she is instructed to do so.

DRUGS FOR PAIN RELIEF

Sedatives and tranquillisers quieten a woman and help her sleep. They are not painkillers. Sometimes they are given in early labour if a woman seems anxious or if things are taking a long time and the midwife considers she needs sleep. If contractions are strong enough to keep you awake they should be actively met and dealt with by controlled breathing and relaxation, and if you are asleep between contractions or in a very drowsy state you cannot do this. As a result you may wake to severe pain which you never manage to get rid of, however hard you struggle to adjust to later contractions.

A woman needs time to adapt herself to labour, and to be led in gently by discovering that she can respond well to early and middle first-stage contractions. If a woman has learned relaxation it will not matter that she is losing sleep, since she is resting, and using only the minimum of energy to adapt herself to contractions. One of the happiest labours I know of lasted three whole days and nights; the woman did not need drugs since she was perfectly relaxed and completely confident, and her partner was with her all the time. But usually long labours are tiring.

One woman was given a sleeping pill when painless contractions were coming at seven-minute intervals at 3.30 a.m. (her baby was not born till the following night at 11.30 p.m.).

She remarked afterwards, 'I wish I had not had the sleeping pill because they started to hurt then and I was too dopey to do anything about it. I kept on coming out of a doze and had more pain than at any other time.'

Epidural and spinal anaesthesia obliterate sensations below the waist but the woman remains conscious.

With regional anaesthesia the woman need neither have general anaesthesia and be 'out for the count', nor be so heavily doped that she is unable to concentrate on breathing and relaxing with contractions. The relatively new types of regional anaesthesia are sometimes spoken of as if they ought to be used for all women in childbirth, regardless of their inclinations, the amount of pain they are feeling, or what they have learned beforehand. Obstetricians often like regional anaesthesia very much because the woman is perfectly controlled and rational, and is in no way overpowered by emotion or by the intensity of the labour experience. She often looks on like a more or less impartial observer of the scene, and he can get on with the task of delivering the baby. It is the sort of situation which fits in well with the routines of a busy hospital, and since the obstetrician frequently has to deliver with forceps or the vacuum-extractor, the delivery can be carefully timed and controlled, and be performed when he is on the spot and ready. Moreover if anything goes wrong with the uterine mechanism or if labour does not start on time, a synthetic form of the hormone oxytocin can be used to initiate and control contractions, without causing any discomfort to the mother. There have been cases of women reading a magazine while the obstetrician worked to deliver the baby down the other end!

But in this very ease of manoeuvre lies a problem. If the woman can feel nothing, or nothing painful, from the waist down, might it not be easier for all concerned if every patient received regional anaesthesia, however early on in labour, or a few days before she was due, with an oxytocin intravenous drip already inserted in her arm, and labour speeded up rapidly so that the obstetrician could be available to deliver at a time suitable for him? This happens often in the USA and increasingly in other countries. But however skilled at delivery the obstetrician is, and however well equipped the hospital with machines which record the baby's every heartbeat, with the instruments which can take a drop of blood from its scalp while still inside the uterus, and devices designed to make birth safer for the baby, patience still remains a virtue in midwifery, and nature is hurried at our peril. For this reason it is probably best to keep regional anaesthesia – which has obvious advantages when the woman has pain which is greater than she can cope with – for cases in which it provides an evident solution to problems which cannot be met by her own responses to uterine stimuli and by emotional support and encouragement.

When an epidural is well sited it removes all pain, and it can even be given so that the woman retains some feeling in her legs, though the so-called 'walking' epidural often proves elusive. In a study of mine, *Some Women's Experiences of Epidurals*,[1] some women said their epidurals were 'pure magic', 'a miracle', and 'like a prayer answered'. 'Within a few minutes I was blissfully numb and it was marvellous. I just can't emphasise enough how wonderful it was to be free of pain and be able to think clearly again.'

But there are side-effects. The woman's blood pressure suddenly drops and she may feel sick and giddy. As one mother put it, 'I experienced a sudden drop in blood pressure and consequently became faint and nauseous. I thought I was about to pass out and die.' This hypotension reduces the oxygen in her blood that is flowing to the baby. So more drugs may be needed to raise her blood pressure again. If your blood pressure is already high a better way of lowering it – and a much gentler method – is to be immersed in water in a birth pool. Research shows that being in warm water is an effective way of reducing blood pressure.

When an epidural has been given contractions may slow down, be less effective, or stop. So labour may be prolonged. Then drugs are given to stimulate the uterus into activity.

The woman has no spontaneous desire to push and must follow instructions. The baby may get stuck in an awkward

---

[1] National Childbirth Trust, 1983.

position because the tone of the pelvic floor muscles has been lost. When the baby's head comes down against the *levator ani* muscles it tends not to rotate to bring the back of the head towards the mother's front. So delivery may have to be assisted with forceps or ventouse. An epidural may result in an instrumental delivery because the baby's head was in the wrong position and pain relief was given because labour was difficult, though if the woman's pushing urge is eradicated by the epidural, and she has no 'birth passion', no spontaneous longing to press the baby through her vagina, this alone is likely to lead to instruments being used to get the baby out.

After-effects may include loss of feeling in the legs for some hours, and inability to empty the bladder for as long as several days, so that a catheter has to be introduced to draw off urine. One woman told me, 'I strongly feel that no mention was made of any possible side-effects by any of the professionals that I consulted and that this was a serious omission on their part.'

An epidural does not always work well either. It may be effective on one side only, not work at all, or even make it difficult to breathe because it is sited too high. When an epidural is one-sided it may feel bizarre and be difficult to cope with, though in my research I found that a few women welcomed the fact that they had still had sensation in the lower part of their bodies. Sometimes the needle penetrates the dura (a thin membrane surrounding the spinal cord) and the drug goes into the space around the spine. Then a much higher dose than was intended is received. The result is, in fact, spinal anaesthesia. From there the drug can enter the cerebro-spinal fluid. After the birth the woman may have the worst headache she ever had in her life, and cannot lift her head from the pillow. Women to whom this happened say, 'After twenty-four hours a headache started which went on for six days', 'I had violent headaches and a dreadful pain in my neck'. Occasionally a woman has difficulty in passing urine, 'I had numbness in the bladder region for about four months'. Or she is left with numb patches or tingling, 'I have had intermittent tingling in my feet and occasional numb toes', 'Twelve months later I still get numbness at the bottom of my spine'. And one woman told me that she had lost sensation in her clitoris, 'I waited patiently after the birth for things to return to normal, but the exquisite intensity of feeling never returned.' The chances of anything like this happening, perhaps in the hands of a less experienced anaesthetist, have to be weighed against the testimony of women who say, 'I thank God I wasn't having babies before epidurals were invented.'

Some women want an epidural because in this way they feel they can co-operate with the birth process without having any discomfort. This is certainly true, but they may not realise that they are also missing something – the intense and thrilling sensations of the descent of the baby's head, which can be not only painless, but enormously satisfying and enjoyable, even though at the same time it feels so extraordinary. Many women do not realise, because the obstetrician did not feel it important to tell them, that with epidurals there is more or less complete *vaginal anaesthesia*. Again and again I have heard women describe the keen sensuous pleasure they obviously experienced – and which often surprised them. It is not a question of just feeling the contractions and knowing when to push, but of the gradual opening up of the vagina like the uncurling petals of a rose. It may look as if it must be traumatic from the other end, and probably a good many of those attending in the delivery room are convinced that it must be painful for all women, and those who do not show it are simply the ones with better self-control; but this is not so. It can bring positive enjoyment, and precedes the sensations of delivery rather as intense sexual pleasure builds up to release in orgasm, and this even when it involves some pain.

Only you can decide. Do not be influenced by what the midwife says she would do in your position. This is your body, your baby and your birth. Bear in mind that, paradoxically, women who choose to have an epidural to maintain or regain control often find that this choice entails other interventions that make them feel out of control.

Gas-and-oxygen is available in the UK for all mothers who want it. It can be taken by the mother herself, who places the mask over her face and inhales through her mouth. Often there is a hole over which she must keep her thumb in order to get the effects of the gas, and as soon as she becomes unconscious her hand slips away and she automatically takes no more. A small quantity of gas-and-oxygen acts mainly as a relaxant and is useful for this purpose. Taken in large amounts, it feels as if you are swimming in treacle – or rather, dreaming of swimming in treacle. Some people feel as if they are floating to the ceiling. Others just feel a warm drowsiness stealing over them.

Analgesics blunt pain and reactions vary; the same amount that makes one woman feel as if she had slightly too much to drink makes another pass out. Pethidine, with gas-and-oxygen the most commonly used obstetric analgesic agent in Britain, is injected into the thigh. If given too early it tends to slow down labour or even to stop it. It may interfere with the baby's breathing at birth, too, and can make breastfeeding more difficult. Mothers who used pethidine in labour tend to jog their babies, to tickle and flick their feet in an attempt to keep them awake for feeding, and this effect on the relationship between a mother and her baby can be long lasting.[2] Pethidine should never be given routinely, and only ever with the woman's consent and understanding of its side-effects.

It is the custom to give pethidine towards the end of the first stage. If a woman has enough of the drug to make any significant difference to her pain she is soon in a stupor, feels drunk, may talk at random, and finds it impossible to synchronise her breathing with contractions. Some women dislike this intensely, and have worse pain than when they are wide awake, controlling their breathing and having their backs rubbed.

The risks of pethidine have been known for a very long time, but it continues to be used without discretion. Writing as far back as 1975, Professor Keiran O'Driscoll[3] cited the following disadvantages: 'nausea, vomiting, disorientation, and mental confusion which leads to failure to co-operate, especially in the second stage of labour'. These disadvantages probably outweigh the advantages of pain relief for most women. He claims that

---

[2] Martin Richards, 'Obstetric Analgesics and the Development of Children', *Midwife, Health Visitor and Community Nurse*, Feb 1976.

[3] *British Journal of Anaesthetics* 47, 1053 (1975).

'many of the discomforts attributed to labour are, in practice, the result of pethidine', and says, 'Labour can be transformed easily into a nightmare experience by pethidine, after which the mother may remain unaware that her baby is born and may suffer a profound sense of depression which continues into the next day.' This is strong language to use about a drug which is freely prescribed in increasingly large doses. When it was first introduced, doctors were advised to use 25 or 50 milligrams. Now it is common practice for it to be given in 100 or 150 mg doses, and since it is offered every three hours or so, many women must be getting 500 mg.

In my own research[4] on 838 reports of their experiences of childbirth written by women who had attended antenatal classes, I found that many described the effects of pethidine as unpleasant, particularly when they felt that they were forced to take it. They said that the rest of labour was 'a complete haze', that they went into a 'stupor', were 'nearly asleep', or had completely lost consciousness for the delivery. Some described ways in which pethidine was given without their consent, and regretted it very much. *When they had choice as to when and if to accept pain relief the effects were much more likely to be good*, and they were more likely to say that 'it took the edge off contractions' or helped them relax.

Perhaps one of the important elements in the study of the effects of drugs on human beings is to discover the circumstances in which they were given, and whether the person taking the drug was happy about taking it, or whether she felt bound to do what she was told. It is very rarely that human considerations such as these are taken into account when effects are analysed.

From these mothers' labour reports, it emerged that when pethidine was given by a midwife with whom the woman had a good relationship, a small dose was often sufficient. It looked as if, in fact, analgesic drugs were sometimes used in place of good emotional support in labour. When there was under-

---

[4] See Sheila Kitzinger, *Some Mothers' Experiences of Induced Labour*, National Childbirth Trust, 1975.

standing support from midwives, this took the place of – and was much more effective than – pharmacological pain relief. This is one good reason why the loving help of a labour companion who can be there all the time and be *depended* on, and who communicates well with the staff, is so important.

There comes a time in most labours when a woman needs someone to breathe *with* her, to say in the middle of a difficult contraction, 'Yes, you're doing it. You're doing beautifully. Good!', to give unstinted praise when she is tired and despairing and perhaps to ask, 'Do you think you can manage just one more contraction?' If she says she can it may be the right time to tell her that she need only handle one contraction at a time, and that if she can manage one more she is doing fine. Each brings nearer the birth of the baby, and that particular contraction will never, ever, come back again.

To give support of this kind is tiring, but exciting and rewarding work. It means sharing what the mother is feeling and being right in there with her, holding her, fixing her attention with your eyes, loving her and *enjoying* the whole adventure of birthing.

Anything that tends to lower the woman's threshold of discrimination means that she may feel out of control. You may decide that you want nothing that a car driver would not take before setting out on a night journey in fog, or an athlete before taking part in a race.

Just as you would not attempt to drive a vehicle while semi-conscious or under the influence of powerful drugs, so you may not want to attempt the important business of having a baby in a doped state. Marjorie Karmel in her book *Babies Without Tears*[5] describes how she was told in an American hospital that the effect of analgesia she would be given was simply that of having one Martini too many. She decided that she did not want to give birth to her child in that state.

Only you can know if you really must have analgesia. You have not failed if you decide to take it. It has been your decision based on your personal experience, and is the right one for you.

---

[5] Secker and Warburg, 1959.

HOW A PARTNER CAN HELP

Throughout labour, support from your partner, or maybe a woman birth companion, is as important as all the preparations. It is not only fear that can lead to the tension which results in pain (Dick-Read's fear-tension-pain syndrome). So can worry that everything is not going according to plan and conflict with the attendants. *Any feeling of frustration can interfere with relaxation and rhythmic breathing*. There should be no talking by anyone in the room during contractions. The best plan is for your birth companion to deal with anything that needs arranging with the doctor or midwife, and with explanations that may be required about the breathing or positions and movements you use. Usually midwives and obstetricians will allow a woman to try things her way and say why they consider that another course of action is necessary, *if a birth companion – either the father or another woman – is present*.

A birth companion should not desert the woman, and leaves her only when and if she can carry on happily for a short time. Sometimes a member of staff will suggest that a birth companion goes out for a cup of tea, or a breath of fresh air, or somewhere quiet to doze off. He or she may return only to find that the woman's morale has dropped, labour has been stimulated with drugs, or she has been persuaded to have pethidine or an epidural.

THE OPENING UP OF THE CERVIX

The whole first stage of labour is concerned with the opening up of the mouth of the uterus. The bands of longitudinal muscle fibre in the main part of the uterus are contracting whilst the cervix is gradually drawing up and apart, and its walls become thinner (see diagrams, pp. 171–5). No voluntary effort can help this process. We have seen that midwives speak of the cervix as one to ten centimetres dilated – ten centimetres being full dilatation, when the cervix is completely effaced, and becomes part of the uterus; uterus, cervix and vagina then form one canal. Some women are already two or three centimetres dilated when they go into labour, dilatation having started without their being aware of it. In most primiparae the cervical canal has already been shortened and the walls drawn up during the three or four weeks before labour begins. In multiparae (women having their second and subsequent babies) the cervix is not usually taken up beforehand.

Dilatation is slowest during the first half of the process. That is, it usually takes a good deal longer to go from one to five centimetres dilatation than to go from five centimetres to full dilatation. Dilatation usually takes between eight to twelve hours or

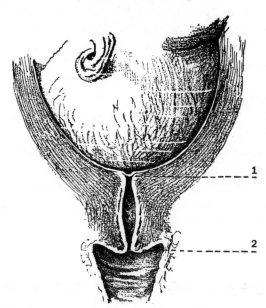

The State of the Cervix at Thirty-Six Weeks in a Primipara

1. Internal os (opening of cervix into uterus)
2. External os

The cervical canal is stopped up with a plug of mucus. During the last month of pregnancy in a woman having her first baby contractions of the upper uterine segment gradually draw up the tissues of the cervix and lower uterine segment. The cervical canal thus gets shorter and shorter until the cervix is of the same thickness as the uterine wall. The cervix is now said to be 'taken up' or 'ripe' for labour. In a multipara the cervix is often not taken up until labour begins.

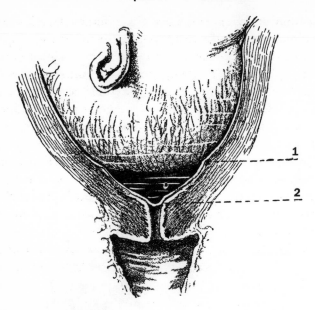

Taking Up of the Cervix

1. Internal os
2. Membranes bulging
The cervical canal has been reduced in length.

more in primiparae, although they are not always aware of the beginning, and between six and ten hours in multiparae. But I have known primiparae who have had a first stage lasting twenty-four hours or more (in some cases without pain), and my first child was born in two and a half very pleasant hours, with some eight to ten painful contractions at the end of the first stage.

Once labour is really under way a woman usually wants someone with her all the time, and she should not be left alone. As each contraction comes it feels like a wave gathering in the distance. She automatically adjusts her breathing rhythm to meet it and as it comes towards her she 'swims' above it with careful, deliberate, rhythmic strokes, right up to the crest; then she begins to feel it fade away and her breathing becomes softer, and she rests. At the end of each contraction she takes a few deep breaths in and out.

Until contractions are coming at five-minute intervals or less full chest breathing is usually sufficient to enable the mother to maintain conscious control over them and it is as well not to use lighter, shallower breathing until, and unless, she really needs to do so. As she breathes in softly and slowly she feels her ribs spread out sideways, the whole bony cage expanding and the sternum lifted, and she continues this breathing steadily throughout each contraction. The woman herself does not feel the beginning of each contraction, although her partner may do so with a hand placed lightly on her abdomen, and can help her be ready for the next contraction by telling her when one is about to come. It is important to begin rhythmic breathing before the height of the contraction is reached.

Empty the bladder regularly throughout labour and remember to go to the lavatory, whether or not you feel you want to,

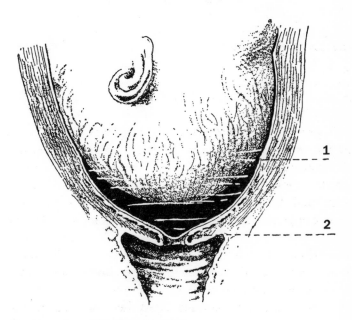

The Cervix Completely Taken Up

1. Internal os
2. Membranes bulging
This shows the state of the cervix early in labour. The canal has disappeared and some dilatation has already taken place.

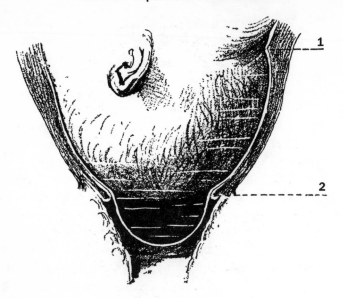

Partial Dilatation of the Cervix in a Primipara

1. Internal os
2. External os

This cervix is about half dilated. The intact bag of waters (the membranes) can be seen bulging through the cervix into the vagina.

every hour or so. A distended bladder can cause acute discomfort as there is pressure against the cervix from the overfull bladder.

The midwife will tell you how far your cervix is dilated after each vaginal examination. You may be eager to be examined because you want to know how you are doing. On the other hand, if you do not want to be examined, a skilled midwife can tell how labour is progressing from the way you look and breathe, and what you are doing during contractions, and you can decline vaginal examinations if you wish. From four or five centimetres dilatation relaxation between contractions as well as during them is essential, and particularly release of the muscles of your abdomen and pelvic floor. When you are ten centimetres dilated your cervix is completely drawn up, and the second stage is about to begin.

Ask the midwife about anything you do not understand at

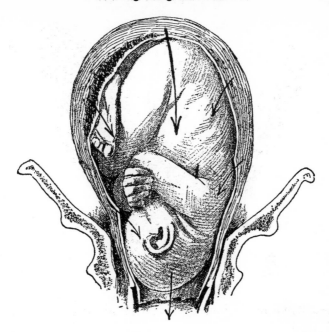

Full Dilatation of the Cervix

Full dilatation of the cervix occurs when it is sufficiently dilated to allow the presenting part, normally the head, but sometimes the buttocks (or breech), to pass through. The membranes have ruptured and the mother is now in the second stage. She is helping the contractions to press the baby down the birth canal.

this, or any other, stage of labour. The advantages of having previously discussed with the midwife your priorities and the kind of labour you hope to have are self-evident.

In spite of the fact that the rate of Caesareans has tripled in the last 25 years, and that obstetricians have become highly expert at doing them, there are strong reasons for avoiding one if possible. Besides the risk of haemorrhage, the likelihood of infection afterwards, the chance that another body organ may be nicked by the scalpel, and loss of muscle tone because muscles have been cut through, even a straightforward Caesarean is a surgical operation from which a woman needs time to recover, just when she has a new baby. She is usually warned that she should not drive or pick up anything heavy for six weeks. The next birth is more likely to be a Caesarean, too,

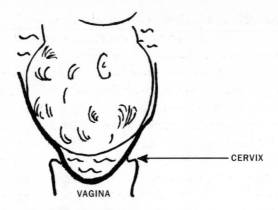

CERVIX

VAGINA

The Membranes Before Rupturing

In the first stage the membranes are usually pressed down through the cervix by the baby's head. They help to dilate the cervix and cushion the baby's head. It is unwise to rupture the membranes artificially until the cervix is at least half dilated, not only because the membranes dilate the cervix evenly, but because they protect the baby's head, and the bubble of amniotic fluid offers a sterile environment. ARM (artificial rupture of the membranes) enables infection to enter, and the more vaginal examinations are done, the more infection is likely. It is for this reason that ARM is a step that, once taken, may mean that labour is artificially accelerated with drugs so that the baby can be born within a set time limit, and that this entails a forceps or ventouse delivery, or even a Caesarean section.

and she has become high risk because she now has a scar in her uterus. It may also be harder to conceive again because of pelvic infection or damage to the endometrium, the lining of the uterus, or the fallopian tubes.

The midwife is there as a skilled friend who can with an experienced eye watch for signs of the progress of labour, interpret them for the parents and help the mother to co-operate fully with the birth process in the way for which she has prepared herself. If the woman has discussed her birth plan and does not confront her as an adversary, the midwife is almost invariably willing to co-operate in achieving the sort of birth she desires. Her name derives from the Anglo-Saxon 'a helping woman' – and that is what she is.

At any time during the first stage the membranes leak, or rupture and shoot out, sometimes with a pop; they feel like a warm, half-set jelly. Rarely they drop down and protrude from the vagina without bursting, and look like a balloon heavy with liquid. There is up to a litre of colourless amniotic fluid inside them. When they are ruptured naturally or by the midwife, *be prepared for an increase in the activity of the contractions immediately after.* They will get stronger and much more efficient and the intervals between them will probably get less. This is because the baby's head presses down more forcefully on the cervix.

You may find that to keep your breathing above the contractions you want to lift your breathing higher. Be prepared to adapt to the new rhythm quickly. There may be a short period during which you do not adapt well, but do not give way to despair. Persevere to keep careful control over the breathing and you will then find the right rhythm and type of breathing to meet these contractions.

Occasionally labour begins and seems to be going well, and then suddenly stops. The mother, who has adjusted herself to the idea of being in labour, is rather perturbed. After half an hour or an hour with nothing at all happening apart from some occasional twinges of backache and a heavy feeling in the pit of her stomach perhaps, she begins to wonder whether she is going to be stuck like this for days.

If this happens and you are not yet half dilated, go for a walk, breathing deeply as you swing your arms rhythmically. Wear two sanitary pads just in case the membranes rupture, and, of course, go with someone who can get you home if labour suddenly starts to speed up.

When you come in, or in any case if the weather is not suitable for a walk, have a warm, scented, luxurious bath and bask in it, but do not lock the door.

Very often a pause of this kind comes before a sudden resumption of activity in the form of the waters bursting and the onset of late first-stage contractions.

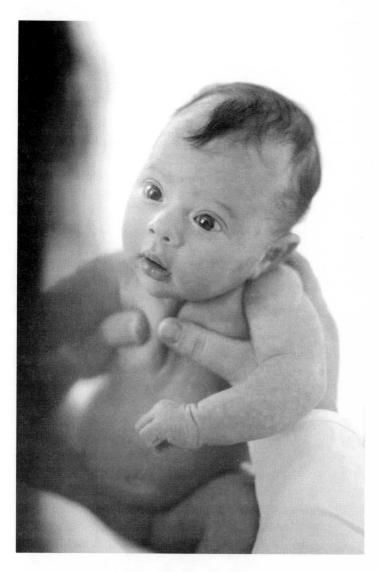

**A newborn baby is a person from the very beginning
and can communicate long before there is speech.**

8

The Climax of Labour

'Is it beyond thee to be glad with the gladness of this rhythm? To be tossed and lost and broken in the whirl of this fearful joy?'

Rabindranath Tagore, *Gitanjali*, lxx.

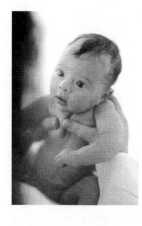

THE END OF THE FIRST STAGE

Contractions are at their most fast and furious between two-thirds dilatation and the end of the first stage. The sensations are strong, overpowering, and can be at the same time delightful. You are swept away like a little boat at sea in a great storm of exultant emotions and a tremendous sweep of physical energy. The body takes over in a marvellous way. It kneads and squeezes; contraction follows contraction powerfully and with precision. In spite of the strength and relentless force of its action there is a delicate accuracy about its workings at this time. You can only be in awe and deliver yourself over, in faith, to this wonderful thing – your body at the work of creation.

It is extremely difficult to describe adequately what a woman in labour feels. I have tried to describe my personal sensations. Most women would probably say that these were painful for at any rate part of this time, but mothers I have prepared for childbirth usually remark: 'but not impossibly uncomfortable', or 'quite bearable', or say that they could 'keep on top of the contractions' with their breathing. Women interpret these sensations in such different ways that whereas one mother will say calmly, 'I did have pain, but it was nothing to speak of, and I felt quite happy', another will seek words to express these sensations by saying, 'It wasn't at all painful. It felt as if I had a warm fire inside me. I could feel a glow as each contraction came,' and still another will feel so glad that at last she is in labour that she will remark, 'It hurt, but it didn't matter.'

As a woman approaches two-thirds dilatation she may start to shiver uncontrollably, and she may vomit. The shivering can be lessened, at any rate, by warm coverings, hot water bottles, perhaps an electric heating pad (covered with a waterproof fabric) and socks. A woman is especially liable to vomit if she has eaten more than light snacks once dilatation has really started. She can often avoid sickness by taking only sips of sweet liquids when labour is definitely under way, but it is important she does not starve herself, because she needs energy, and if she is hungry she may enjoy bread and honey, banana, soup, ice-cream, a smoothie, or an egg dish – anything that she fancies really.

Except in fog or very cold weather, or when a premature baby is expected, it is as well to leave the windows open until delivery is imminent, as the fresh air is good. Move around, be upright as much as possible, and change position until you are comfortable. You may want to be in different positions and swing, rock, tilt and circle your pelvis. During the late first stage you will probably need helping in doing this as you may feel very heavy and almost fixed to the bed. You can lean against furniture or be well supported with pillows or a beanbag so that you can relax in comfort. Even if your midwife would prefer you to labour in bed because it is more convenient for her, you don't have to. Women are sometimes told that they must stay on the bed because that is the only way the baby's heart can be monitored, or even because the floor is dirty. You can say that you would like the heart monitored intermittently with a sonic aid. This means that you can be mobile except when the heart is being checked. If the floor is dirty it should be cleaned. Offer to mop it yourself if necessary! It would be a good way to move.

Contractions get stronger and stronger and appear to have a reckless intensity, the intervals between them growing shorter until they are down to two minutes or less. They bring with them acute abdominal tension and you feel rather as if an enormous balloon was being blown up inside and then slowly deflated.

You may have lifted your breathing higher and be doing quick breathing at the height of each contraction now. It comes much more easily than when you were practising it during pregnancy. At the end of each contraction breathe deeply and rest completely, and use the interval between contractions to centre down and be sure that you are really relaxed.

The midwife may want to examine you vaginally every now and then to see how far the opening of the uterus is dilated. The cervix hangs like the clapper of a bell inside the birth canal, so she can feel it with her fingers. She should let you know the progress you are making. It is not sufficient to make what one mother complained of as merely 'soothing noises'. This examination need not hurt at all, especially if you remember to relax and after taking a deep breath, breathe out whilst the midwife inserts her gloved fingers, and at the same time release the muscles of the pelvic floor.

It is better not to be examined during a contraction, as you want to concentrate on it and are too preoccupied. If the midwife attempts examination during a contraction ask her to wait a moment, or your birth companion should be alert to request this. If you keep your eyes open you can easily indicate by shaking your head or lifting your hand that you would prefer her to wait a minute.

You can be examined in the left lateral position, which entails lying in the front lateral with your face to the left, drawing up your left leg towards your breast and rounding your back.

Obstetricians and midwives often prefer you in a dorsal or modified lithotomy position for examination. In this case lie on your back with your legs apart and knees bent. In the true lithotomy position your legs are raised in stirrups. Some women find that they suffer from painful cramp in the legs, or are terribly uncomfortable, in the lithotomy position. In this case, say so. If you have pain in your thighs, it can be relieved by either gentle or very firm massage up and down your upper legs from the pelvis and back to it again. Either you or your birth companion can do this. If pain is centred around your pubis and groin, at the very base of your abdomen, you can do very light massage, using the fleshy pads of your fingers with a circular rhythmic movement.

It is important that however drowsy you may feel *between* contractions – and this drowsiness is nature's way of achieving muscular release – you *greet each contraction with your breathing* and harmonise with the contraction wave.

Sometimes a woman feels disconcertingly cut off from reality, and hates the feeling. It is rather as if you were in a spaceship and had lost contact with earth, with none of the usual points of reference, in a timeless, limitless existence. It is exacerbated by loneliness, isolation and the monotony of continually recurring contractions in a long-drawn-out labour. Some women happily accept this sensation of drift, but others fight against it.

A condition known as *kayak-angst* has been described among Eskimos. When the Eskimo hunter is out alone on a calm sea paddling or sitting quietly, there develops a lowering in the level of consciousness brought on by the absence of external reference points at a time when the hunter is engaged in simple repetitive movements or sitting motionless, and staring at the sea. He gets confused and dizzy – and even the psychologists who were studying this found that they were disturbed in exactly the same way when they tried to do it, too.

This condition may arouse vivid memories in some women who have been alone in a hospital labour ward for any length of time, lying with nothing to see but the ceiling and a tiled wall, sometimes with a light shining in their faces.

The situation in labour is, of course, rather different, because the effect of stimulatory deprivation (through loneliness, silence, postural immobility, confinement in a small room, bare surroundings, often unpatterned and clinically white walls) is coupled with intense stimulation from one organ of the body, the contracting uterus. In such cases the result can be a failure of nerve.

It is important to create points of reference to avoid this sort of stress that threatens a woman's equilibrium. The labouring woman should not be left alone unless she wishes it, and should wear glasses if she requires them. Familiar objects, the presence of her partner or a midwife or doctor she already knows and likes, the use of phrases she is familiar with to help her remember what she has learned and to keep relaxed control, and reference to the preparation she has received, so that she is reminded that she has rehearsed it all before, can help. When she feels shivery, or says that she does not want her baby today, or wants to go home now, or that she just needs to sleep and forget her labour, she should have someone there to remind her that these are all normal occurrences in a labour that is going well, and are, in fact, signs of progress.

TRANSITION BETWEEN FIRST AND SECOND STAGES

Gradually you feel the contractions change. They become irregular, and you get a catch in your throat at their height. You realise that this is the expulsive reflex, though you may not be fully dilated and should not push voluntarily. While you can still ask whether you should push, you are not yet ready to do so. Only when the desire to bear down is *completely irresistible* do you start pressing the baby down the birth canal. It may take quite a long time – half an hour or more. Whether or not you deliberately decide to push the baby out by your own exertions, it will get born.

You may get irritable and want to 'get away from it all'. Women sometimes protest, 'Oh, do go away and leave me alone' or 'I only want to sleep', or get bad-tempered.

A slight and natural developing amnesia is often further reinforced by opiate drugs and then it is usually much more difficult to control the impulse towards flight by conscious and positive redirection of your thoughts, by making the decision to enter into your labour rather than to try and avoid it. This is one of the reasons why opiates create difficulties and are not a solution to the problem of pain in labour.

If you seem to be escaping into a dream world – which is more one of nightmare than being overwhelmed by the creative power in your body – it is important that your birth companion should bring you back to reality with stimulation. He can wring out face cloths or sponges in very cold, preferably iced, water and rest them against your forehead, cheeks, lips and the nape of your neck with each contraction. As you are probably feeling rather sticky and hot by now this is refreshing. Your birth companion can help you move into a more comfortable position and swing and rock your pelvis, too.

Some women, especially those whose babies are in an occipito-posterior position, have severe backache during this phase. While massage often relieves it, you may be most comfortable on all fours, with your legs and arms apart, taking the weight of the baby off your spine, and resting it on the front of your pelvis, and rocking the pelvis slightly forwards and back during a contraction. Some women like firm, regular massage of the adductors (the muscles of the inner thigh). This is of particular help if it is difficult to relax your legs because you get 'shivery'. If your legs jerk during contractions, or if you curl up your toes, your legs are not completely relaxed. Very rarely the cord prolapses when the baby's presenting part is high. Then it is important to relieve pressure on it by allowing the baby's head or whichever part is presenting to fall well away from the bony rim of the pelvis between contractions. The midwife may suggest that you kneel leaning forward with your knees near your chest, if this happens.

This is the point in labour when you may forget that you are having a baby. Your partner can remind you that before very long you will be holding the baby in your arms. This is one of the most difficult phases of labour, but it rarely lasts more than about half an hour and soon you will be able to push the baby out.

Some women start gasping as the contraction reaches its height. In this case, quickly blow out and start breathing rhythmically again. It helps if your partner is close to you and breathes with you to give moral support. A woman who has been doing shallow rapid breathing with her lips apart for some time always requires a drink, or at any rate a sip of water to moisten her dry lips and mouth. She can have a little raspberry leaf tea, tea, coffee or fruit juice, or, if she is feeling sick, iced water. Many women cannot digest fruit squash at this time. A few sips of strong, black, sugary coffee particularly will act as a stimulant and may help her if she is beginning to feel that her labour is 'getting on top' of her. But she should not drink so much that her bladder becomes distended, as this can slow up labour by creating a sort of traffic jam inside her.

The urge to push often comes very suddenly and over-whelmingly.

Sometimes the rim of the cervix fails to retract equally all round the advancing head, and a part of it – at the front – is caught up over the baby's head for a few minutes, or occasionally longer. This is known as 'an anterior lip'. It is particularly common with posterior presentations.

Continued forceful pushing against an incompletely dilated cervix can make it puffy and swollen so that the opening, instead of getting wider for the baby's head to come through, is made smaller and labour is held up. The best thing to do is to stop pushing (if you can) and wait patiently for full dilatation. But if you have to push, you have to push! If the urge to do so is overwhelming you need not wait for anyone to give you permission to bear down. Your body knows what to do.

You will hear your breathing becoming rather noisy. This noisier breathing is perfectly natural and *is not an indication that you are in pain*. If you keep your chin well forward on your chest you will sound less desperate.

THE SECOND STAGE

First baby: 'This stage . . . was not painful at all even when the head crowned. My husband sat at the head of the bed with his arms round my waist to support me. I was very comfortable. I was not in the least tired. There was no pain at all. I could feel the baby's head behind the rectum like a very hard lump. Be-tween contractions I was so completely relaxed that I could not

answer when anyone spoke to me. I know I was using the contractions well and the midwives remarked on this and how well
I relaxed.'

First baby: 'I began really to enjoy the birth. It was a wonderful thing to be able to use the power of the contractions to make
the baby come. I suppose I have never worked with such a sense
of power and assurance of success . . . A most satisfying and
rewarding experience.'

First baby: 'It was the most wonderful work, but very hard.
My husband soon could see the head.' The midwife insisted on
her taking gas-and-oxygen and placed the mask on her face,
'but I kept pushing it away, saying, "No, thank you; I have no
pain. I have no use for that." I don't think I would have enjoyed
the birth so much with it.'

First baby: 'I had no analgesia, and it was just a case of hard
work.'

Second baby, after a very painful first labour. 'The second stage
was easy. Two magnificent pushes – no wasted effort there.'

First baby: 'I certainly felt completely unafraid and look back
on it as the most wonderful experience imaginable . . . The
second stage was completely happy and painless.'

First baby: 'I can honestly say I felt no actual pain, though I
had slight backache.'

First baby, at onset of second stage: 'Oh, isn't this exciting?'

First baby, high forceps delivery with spinal anaesthesia: 'The
doctor nicked the rim of my cervix and the baby was delivered
by forceps. My husband saw her born, and particularly enjoyed
watching her uncurling as she came out of the birth canal. He
told me her sex. I was very excited and felt nothing of the birth
except a sensation of pulling during the delivery.'

Third baby: 'I thought I could feel the wedge of waters pushing its way down the birth canal, and simultaneously the strong
urge to push. The midwife ruptured the waters, whereupon the
head pressed on the perineum and she asked me to pant. The
rapid shallow breathing came easily. The next push produced
the baby's head.'

First baby (a trial of labour in which everything was in readi-
ness for Caesarean section if necessary. The mother, however,

gave birth to the baby spontaneously): 'It was marvellous, it was such a beautiful rhythm. G. [her husband] sloshed cold water on my face in between contractions. He had his arm behind my head and held it forward for each contraction. I had oxygen and that was a great help.'

The second stage is that of the expulsion of the baby. The arc through which the baby travels in its journey through the birth canal is shown in the diagram. Women often enjoy it, and the pleasure it brings is similar to a small child's simple delight in defecation. When the bearing-down reflex is fully established the urge to push is compelling and irresistible. Some women are horrified at the intensity of the desire to bear down. 'It is', as one mother commented afterwards, 'a very primitive sort of urge. I was astonished that it was so strong.' Women who are not prepared for the passion they feel welling up in them may try to escape from the sensations. They panic and grip themselves in pain, resisting the urge with all their might.

The second stage need not be at all painful. It is often pleasurable even for unprepared women who can enjoy co-ordinated muscular effort. If you are not pushed beyond your powers by over-enthusiastic attendants who take on the role of cheerleaders, rather than patiently and quietly standing by, there is

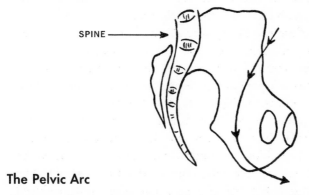

SPINE

The Pelvic Arc

This diagram illustrates the movement of the baby down into and through the pelvis during labour. Very often the baby has entered the pelvis some weeks before labour starts. Note that the descent and expulsion is not in a straight line, but in a gentle curve. Visualise this arc when you are bearing down during the second stage.

no reason why, if you know what to expect and trust your body, it should be anything but exhilarating and very satisfying. Gas-and-oxygen is unnecessary, although it is sometimes taken by women who felt they needed it for the transition phase between the first and second stages but continue to take it, 'from habit', or because they are 'scared', and not because they are in pain, as they admit afterwards.

There are no rules about the position in which you give birth. Though your doctor or midwife may be accustomed to catching babies with women propped up on their backs, you may want to squat, kneel, half-squat half-kneel, be on all fours, or lean forward from a standing or kneeling position, holding on to furniture, the bedhead or your partner.

If you cannot get pushing quite right, you will almost invariably be able to do so if you squat, kneel or half-squat half-kneel and push in that position. In most traditional birth cultures women have their babies in this way. The pelvis is at its widest when the mother is upright with knees bent. It is hard to think of any position that makes birth more difficult than lying on your back, except for lying on your back with your legs in the air. This is the lithotomy position, often used in hospitals. The woman lies with her buttocks at the edge of the delivery table, for the convenience of the obstetrician, with her knees pulled back towards her body and her legs constrained in stirrups. These are set wide apart so that there is a large working area for the obstetrician. When a woman is on her back the baby must come up rather than down. Instead of having gravity to help her, she has to fight against it. If her legs are in stirrups terrific pressure is put on her perineum, too, so that it is more likely to tear. Stirrups may cause venous thrombosis by exerting pressure on blood vessels in her legs and also reduce the oxygen supply to the baby.

Roberto Caldeyro-Garcia, an obstetrician with deep understanding of the physiology of normal birth, who was President of the International Federation of Obstetricians and Gynaecologists, used to say that the supine position for labour and birth is the worst possible except for being hung by the feet.

It was generally accepted through most of the twentieth

century that this was a time of enormous effort and muscular straining, and the classic picture of a woman in the second stage of labour was that of the mother grunting and groaning with effort, sweat streaming off her face, veins standing out on her forehead, lips pressed together, eyes glazed and skin red and hot, while her cheer-leading attendants exhorted her to still further efforts. Women were told that they must work hard, that this was an athletic achievement which demanded strength and persistence, and that they would feel tired out after the birth. Even in otherwise easy labours, women were exhausted; their lips were parched, their eyes bloodshot; they felt weak and once the baby was born only wanted to be left alone to sleep.

So intimately was the idea of physical exertion associated with childbirth that some midwives used to urge the mother to push, to 'lean on the pains', long before she desired to, and before her cervix was effaced, putting extreme stress on the transverse cervical ligaments, which often were torn, and sometimes produced an oedematous cervix through which the baby's head could not pass easily. This resulted in a delayed second stage, an episiotomy and sometimes a high forceps delivery. The pushing stage was a formidable display of strenuous effort. The woman felt desperate and her actions became uncoordinated. She lost trust in her body and simply struggled to follow commands. If this happened when we were trying to empty our bowels we might all need anal episiotomies! More recently it has come to be generally realised that the mother must not push until her body is ready for it, the head can be seen and the way is clear for its expulsion.

The baby's head on the perineum stimulates an urge referred to medically as 'Ferguson's reflex'. If you have had an epidural you probably won't feel this. Then it makes sense to push when you know that the head is on the perineum, but not earlier, because this can be harmful and actually delay the birth.

Pushing before the physiological stimulus builds up is counterproductive. You waste energy and become exhausted if you push for a long time, and tissues get swollen as a result of friction, so that instead of opening wider, they close up.

Even now some midwives and obstetricians want to get the

baby born as soon as possible once the second stage has really started, even when there are no signs of fetal distress, and exhort the woman to push harder and longer. If she shows no signs of wanting to push, she is often told, 'Just try a little one, dear, and see what happens.'

If you have been pushing to order, see what happens if you stop pushing and just let the contractions wash over you, breathing your way through them. This gives your body a chance to

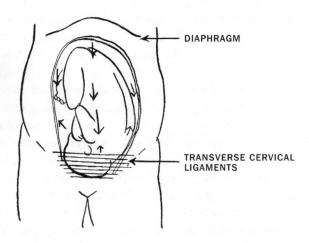

DIAPHRAGM

TRANSVERSE CERVICAL
LIGAMENTS

Diagram showing the effect of uterine contractions acting alone with minimum straining by the mother.

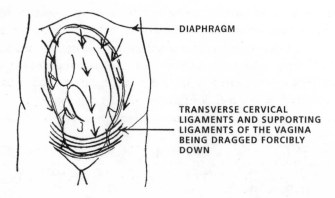

DIAPHRAGM

TRANSVERSE CERVICAL
LIGAMENTS AND SUPPORTING
LIGAMENTS OF THE VAGINA
BEING DRAGGED FORCIBLY
DOWN

Diagram showing the effect of bearing down while the cervix is insufficiently dilated, or when the vagina is still tight.

get into the natural rhythm again, for the swelling to subside, the baby's head to be eased down by the power of the uterus alone, and the spontaneous reflex to push to build up.

The idea of birth as an athletic achievement – the simile drawn is often that of rowing – was popular in the method of *accouchement sans douleur* taught by Fernand Lamaze. Under this system the obstetrician kept up a running commentary on the progress of labour. Though some women liked this constant encouragement, others were distressed by the continual flow of words, the reiterated, '*Alors! Madame, attention! Poussez! Poussez . . . Poussez . . . Poussez . . . Encore! Encore! Continuez! Continuez! . . . Très bien. Très bien. Reposez-vous. Respirez bien.*' etc.[1]

The better the co-ordination of uterine contractions, muscular activity and breathing rhythm, the less effort is required from the woman, and a relaxed and natural second stage results. The important thing to remember is that you should *listen* to contractions to remain sensitive and aware of them, and be alert to any change in their character. The urge to push varies greatly from contraction to contraction. You push exactly when and as long as, and as strongly as, each indicates. It is a little like the orchestra responding to the conductor's baton. The contracting uterus is the conductor.

Constance Beynon's research[2] indicates that babies get born satisfactorily and with less need for forceps deliveries and for episiotomies when the mother economises in muscular effort and is permitted to follow her own inclinations, when 'pushing' is not mentioned by her attendants and she is not hurried at all. Mrs Beynon started her investigations after noting that cardiac cases, who were not allowed to strain in labour, had their babies just as easily as normal healthy patients, and she discovered that the more perfect the co-ordination the less conscious effort was

---

[1] Lamaze made a record of a labour conducted by himself. It is interesting to compare this with the tranquil record of a birth with Dick-Read. The film of a labour conducted by Vellay, *Naissance*, is very beautiful, and much more peaceful than Lamaze's record.

[2] See Constance L. Beynon, 'The Normal Second Stage of Labour', *J. of Obst. and Gynae. of the Br. Emp.*, Vol. LXIV, No. 6, December 1957.

needed and the less expulsive force required, because the resistance presented by the pelvic floor was minimal. Only irresistible pushing was necessary, and only the minimum of that.

A woman who has learned to push using her diaphragm should know that, however conscious, voluntary and controlled her actions when she was practising, in labour this action will come naturally. The point of learning how to do it beforehand is that delicate co-ordination between muscular action and the contractions is necessary in labour, and she is more likely to have full confidence in herself and to trust her own body if she knows what is happening and does not rely upon commands coming from other people, but can interpret her physical sensations and know how to react to them instantaneously, without doubt or hesitation. Moreover, a woman who has learned beforehand the kind of muscular activity she will enjoy in the second stage of labour does not tense up muscles that are not involved in expulsion. She keeps her shoulders rounded forwards, her chin tucked in against her chest, her jaw relaxed, and, above all, the muscles of her pelvic floor released as she pushes, rounding rather than arching her back, and automatically rocking her pelvis forward. After each contraction she relaxes completely.

She steadies herself for each contraction by taking one or two deep breaths as it begins. As it rises towards its height she will know whether or not to push with that one, and whether she must push, but only gently. If it is a powerful one she will find that her breath is held involuntarily and that her ribs and diaphragm become fixed, and she pushes down on her uterus with her diaphragm, and relaxes the abdominal muscles. This pressure comes entirely from above and she does not tighten at all below.

Sometimes the perineum becomes rigid and shiny as the baby's head presses against the pelvic floor. You can slow this down so that your perineum has time to dilate gradually and can take the passage of the baby's head without laceration or an episiotomy, unless for the baby's sake it is essential that it should be born quickly, which happens sometimes. Occasionally uterine contractions in themselves are so strong that

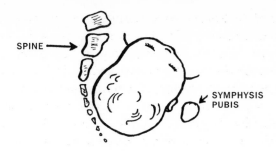

The Descent of the Baby's Head

During the late first and the second stage many women feel severe backache – or they may feel just 'a bump' that moves down with each second stage contraction.

little can be done about it, but push *only when the urge to push is irresistible.* Stop pushing and *pant lightly for the next few contractions and blow out as each reaches its peak,* until the perineum is no longer taut. In this way the birth outlet will probably dilate to allow the birth of the baby's head without a tear.

As the coccyx and sacrum are pushed up and backward by the pressure of the baby's head passing over the pelvic floor you may experience temporary backache and try in vain to adjust your position to get more comfortable. Welcome it, since it means that the baby is already much lower. When the baby's head is posterior backache is likely to be much more severe. You may feel the bump which is the baby's head move down with each contraction and recede again slightly at the end.

You feel the pressure of the baby's head against your rectum as it moves still lower and reaches the deepest point in the arc of its journey. It feels very much like a grapefruit – and indeed has something of this consistency, since the bones of the baby's skull slightly overlap each other at the fontanelles so as to ease its passage into the world. The moulding of the baby's head immediately after birth results from the pressure of the birth canal.

If a woman is pushing hard because she feels this is what is *expected* of her in the second stage, and not because her uterine contractions demand it, or because she senses an atmosphere of haste or urgency, or if she is pushing against an as yet inadequately dilated perineum, the feeling she experiences will be one of extreme discomfort. This cannot always be avoided when the baby is very large.

Although these few moments tend to be quickly forgotten after the birth of the baby, they are not pleasant and many women feel it was the time when their self-control was most threatened. They felt they were 'going to pop' and describe the sensation as 'preposterous'.

As soon as the baby's head crowns – that is, as soon as the tip of it protrudes and does not slip back again – you must be ready to stop pushing, even though you feel like it. Then the head will be born more gently. You may be able to feel or, if you are watching, can see yourself when this happens, and stop. If you are not yet aware that the baby is about to be born – too busy bearing down – or you do not want to look, stop immediately whoever is catching the baby tells you to. You can then look down and catch the first glimpse of your baby.

THE BIRTH

> The morning stars sang together, and all the sons of God shouted for joy.
>
> _The Book of Job_

First baby: 'I felt the baby slide out gently. There was no sensation of splitting – just a gentle opening up. The baby cried. I asked to hold her hand.'

First baby: 'I saw the head when I sat up for the next contraction. That was marvellous. Then the mouth opened very, very wide and he yelled.'

First baby: 'It was wonderful. I had three contractions for which I bore down. John [her partner] helped in delivering her, and she was born screaming.'

First baby: 'The head appeared and I looked down to see it and then another contraction and it was well through. Still no pain or even a feeling of stretching – it just felt rather hard . . . The baby was born and there was still no pain and it was very thrilling to see it being born and hear my husband say it was a girl. She yelled loudly as soon as she was born, and the cord was cut and I held her.'

First baby: 'I could feel her kicking and heard her first cry. It was the most wonderful moment in our lives.'

First baby – on seeing her baby's head ooze out and rotate: 'Oh how adorable! Oh darling, how adorable! It's my baby!'

Third baby: 'Panting made me feel really secure at the crowning. I looked down as the head was being born and heard him cry while his body was still inside me. It was very exciting – for my husband too. He really enjoyed it . . . The baby was laid on my abdomen feeling warm, wet and full of life.'

First baby – the father comments on his daughter's birth: 'I shall never forget the look on her face as the baby slipped out. It was wonderful. Triumph, well-being and joy . . . One could never capture it in a photograph . . . It was the most wonderful experience. It is the sort of thing I shall never forget.'

The crowning is usually believed to be one of the most painful moments of labour, and many women dread it. Some babies' heads do not crown. If the mother is pushing down hard and without sensitivity, ignoring the dictates of her uterus, and if she fails to wait for the gradual dilatation of the perineum, the head may pop out like a cork out of a champagne bottle instead. Her perineum may be torn and repair will be necessary. With the ideal birth, however, the crowning of the head, its birth and the birth of the body all take place slowly and gently.

The woman begins to feel herself gradually opening up, like a bud into full flower, a strange experience which may be rather frightening. This is accompanied by a warm tingling sensation as the baby's head begins to make the perineum bulge forward. The feeling is very acute and some women hate it; they find it shocking. It is a sensation so vivid that they do not know whether it is pleasure or pain, whether to welcome or retreat from it. For some it is almost as if they are being violated, and this can be a particularly difficult moment for women who have ever been sexually abused. The woman who is adequately prepared – both physically and *emotionally* – for the experience of birth, greets these sensations with delight.

Since the head is the largest part of the baby the vulva is

stretched to its widest capacity, and often remains so for several minutes till one, two or three contractions have pushed the whole body out. If the vulva is not dilating naturally the person who is catching the baby may do a quick episiotomy during a contraction, and then the baby's head can slip out easily. But an episiotomy should never be performed routinely. It is a cultural rite of female genital mutilation that has been discredited by research. Student midwives and doctors in teaching hospitals have to do a certain number of episiotomies as part of their training. If you are having your baby in a teaching hospital, it is worth enquiring about that. An episiotomy may be considered necessary because the uterus is pushing the baby down too fast. This can happen when the uterus has been artificially stimulated with drugs. As one woman who had an episiotomy and an assisted delivery told me, 'The labour had been stimulated too fast and baby had type 2 dips (in the heart rate), and I had to have a quick forceps delivery.' It is not just a matter of the size of the baby's head. I know mothers who have had very large first babies and suffered no injury to the perineum. A perineal wound makes a lot of difference to how you feel afterwards. Women say, 'I found the after-effects of the stitches the most draining part of childbirth. I felt full of energy and completely well just after the birth . . . but when my stitches began to hurt I started to feel very tired and limp', 'I found that even after short spells of standing my perineum ached and throbbed' and 'I was still walking with difficulty after a week.' You can imagine how this can affect your sex life. After an episiotomy problems with sexual intercourse often continue for months.[3]

For a woman who is giving birth actively the moment when the head crowns is an intensely pleasurable and very exciting one. Like many other childbirth teachers I used to tell mothers that they would feel 'a splitting, burning sensation', until one

---

[3] Sheila Kitzinger and Penny Simkin (eds), *Episiotomy and the Second Stage of Labor,* 2nd edition 1986, International Childbirth Education Association; Sheila Kitzinger and Rhiannon Walters, *Some Women's Experiences of Episiotomy,* National Childbirth Trust, 2nd edition 1993.

wrote to tell me that she had not felt anything like this and it had been pleasant. After that I described the sensations of bulging without adding any suggestion that the crowning was not to be enjoyed, and since then have discovered that few women have complained about it. In fact, there is no reason why it cannot be a thrilling and very happy part of the birth. There is a high degree of desensitisation of the perineum because of the pressure of the head, and the feeling, though acute, is usually not one of pain but of extreme pressure and heat. When you see the rounded shape of your baby's head and its damp, dark hair you suddenly forget about yourself entirely and are concerned only for your child. The head looks amazingly large, and if you knew nothing about the mechanisms involved you would probably wonder how it was going to get out. It continues to rotate so that it presents the narrowest diameter and can slide out easily. This part of the birth must not be hurried and it is best to allow the baby to be born by uterine contractions without any forcing on your part. If and when the midwife wants you to push or to squeeze gently she will tell you. Otherwise take it for granted that you should *not* be bearing down.

Pant lightly and 'breathe the baby out'. A woman who is lying flat on her back, and hence only partly aware of the birth, may find it very difficult to control herself at this time.

All this time it is very important to relax the muscles of the birth outlet. Actively release them so that you feel as if you are helping the baby's head to bulge through.

The woman feels as if her whole body is becoming a gateway into the world for her child. The head begins to ooze out. She may be asked to squeeze gently *between* contractions to help this process. The gates swing back and open wide. This is the moment of triumph and exaltation. The baby is sliding down. The head is born to below the chin. It may look very blue, even purple. The child has not yet taken the first great gasp of air into its lungs. The practice of routinely suctioning the baby's airways is outmoded and can cause damage to sensitive tissues. If, as sometimes happens, the cord is twisted around the neck, the midwife will unhook it with her finger, or clamp and cut it immediately. First the anterior shoulder is born, and then the other comes out. The baby's warm damp arms rest on the mother's thighs and then the whole body slips out, wriggling and soft. But even before the body is born the chest may flutter and swell and the child may open wide its mouth and cry – a high-pitched wailing scream. The baby suddenly turns red, and the mother gasps with pleasure at this, the first greeting, the first reaction to being thrust into life and out from the warm, swaying comfort of her body. She wants to take the child in her arms immediately to hold him tight and soothe him. The muscles of the little body may seem clenched in protest, in indignation at being born. The mother laughs; he looks so annoyed, so helpless, his rage is so futile, and she wants to protect him from himself and his own violent emotions. Whether boy or girl, she realises that this child is exactly what she desired.

It used to be thought that every baby had to cry at birth, or there was something wrong with it. The Apgar score, by which newborn vigour is assessed, lists a cry, or at least 'a grimace', as one important element in rating vitality, and is still in general use. We know now that a baby need not cry, or may give a startled cry and then settle down to explore the environment. After I wrote the first edition of this book I had another baby and, since I had five hours' intermittent backache and only twenty minutes' active labour, we were not quick enough to call the midwife. Uwe was filming and I wanted him to get a clear picture, so I did not put my hands down, but let the baby creep out by herself. She did not cry, but went pink, crawled up to my breast, rooted around, latched on, and sucked energetically.

You can ask the midwife to wait before clamping the cord for it to stop pulsating so that the baby gets all the blood possible. The fingers of her left hand rest on the cord, her right hand grasping the scissors with which she will cut this gelatinous mass, which is twisted round and round like a malacca cane and sometimes even loosely knotted, evidence of the activity that you felt inside the uterus, and the way in which the baby kicked, bumped, squirmed, twisted, somersaulted, and swam in your body like a fish in the sea. The cord is clamped in two places and cut 10 or 11 cms away from the baby between the two clamps. If you choose to have a physiological third stage, which entails delayed cord clamping – waiting to clamp it until it has stopped pulsating – an injection to stimulate the uterus to expel the placenta should not be given, because when the uterus squeezes down the placenta may get stuck. Active (intrusive) and physiological management of the third stage should not be mixed. The child is now a separate individual.

HOW THE BABY LOOKS

The baby may be covered with a white creamy substance rather like cream cheese which has been protecting the delicate skin *in utero*. This is called *vernix caseosa* and gradually washes off, although it is rarely completely removed at the first bath. Some midwives think this affords valuable protection in the first few days of life and do not attempt to remove it. Sometimes babies have fine hairs all over their skin, the lanugo which also afforded protection *in utero*. You notice it over the baby's arms and in the small of the back and low over the forehead and at the sides of the cheeks. This hair gradually falls out. The first crop of hair on the head usually also disappears to be replaced by a new crop which may be of a different, and often lighter, colour. As this happens some babies look as if they are getting red haired.

Occasionally the membranes have not ruptured over the baby's head and the child is born with a caul like a cap over the vault of the skull or even over the whole head.

The baby who has not been doped by excessive analgesia usually breathes immediately. It is important to breathe as soon as possible after birth, as otherwise there may be damage to brain cells due to lack of oxygen. Between 35 per cent and 67 per cent (according to different research studies done) of babies whose mothers have been doped with opiates do not breathe immediately at birth, whereas only 2 per cent of babies of mothers who have received no analgesia do not breathe immediately. The midwife and obstetrician have various techniques to get the baby to cry, and so to breathe. Usually all that needs to be done is to clear mucus from the airways, and tilt the baby with head lower than the chest so that it drains out. The midwife hands the baby to the mother, who holds her in her arms, marvelling at the perfection of every detail, the tiny shell-pink fingernails and the faint eyelashes and brows. The child clutches her finger firmly in a tight grasp and may go to sleep on her breast.

Meanwhile the afterbirth may have detached itself from the lining of the uterus and slipped into the vagina, waiting to be expelled, or there may be further uterine contractions to deliver it. If the uterus needs help to expel the placenta the midwife may use controlled cord traction. Occasionally the placenta follows the baby right down, and they emerge in one big bundle.

The placenta, red and meaty, is criss-crossed with blood vessels. The midwife examines it and you can ask to see it, too. It has been the tree of life for your baby. The uterus quickly contracts, and hour by hour sinks lower in the mother's body till in ten days or less it is no longer an abdominal but a pelvic organ. After six weeks it is back to its normal state, or, in the case of a first baby, is a little larger than it was before conception.

After the baby is born you will have some discharge. This lochia is evidence that the lining of the uterus is repairing itself. For several days or so it is usually bright red. Then it turns pale pink for a few more days (or sometimes weeks) and finally you may notice it only after a breastfeed. Stimulation of the breasts results in contractions of the uterus. (You may feel these as 'after-pains', which can be uncomfortable.) If you don't lie around, but keep on the move, this lochia will drain from the uterus more rapidly.

AFTER THE BIRTH

The midwife begins to tidy up, while the mother who has been active throughout the birth and who has leaned forward to see her baby born is radiant and transfigured now. Far from feeling tired and worn out, she experiences a glow of health and well-being, and an overwhelming joy. She feels that she has been able to share in the work of creation. She feels love for her partner who has been beside her and has helped her, so that they know that they have done this together, and a great spirit of thanksgiving. As one new mother said, 'I feel swamped with love and affection for the world . . . It is because it was for me – and for H. [her partner] too – so complete an experience that I am so madly in love with the child.' Simone de Beauvoir, in *The Second Sex*, describes the feelings of a woman who must surely have been delivered under anaesthesia, so different are they from the experience of one who has had a natural birth. 'Some women suffer from the emptiness they now feel in their bodies: it seems to them that their treasure has been stolen . . . But just what part has the mother had in the extraordinary event that brings into the world a new existence? She does not know . . . There is an astonished melancholy in seeing him outside, cut off from her. And almost always a disappointment.'

If the birth takes place at home, the midwife leaves, and the couple are left alone with their child. Once they have proudly telephoned the grandparents they are suddenly aware of the peace of being together, the house quiet, with their sleeping child. They are now a family. They have experienced together something incomprehensibly wonderful – a peak of joy in their life which will perhaps always be for them a symbol of the deepest sort of love they know. Their relationship has gained something from this – and through the months of pregnancy and the short space of a few hours in which new life entered the world it acquired a fullness of joy which, whatever their failings and mistakes later, can never be entirely forgotten. Childbirth that is shared by a couple has significance which reaches far beyond the act of birth itself, and through them has its effect upon society.

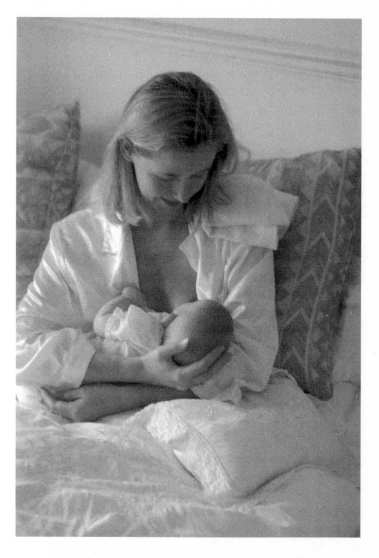

Breastfeeding is not just a matter of filling a baby's tummy with milk, but one element in an evolving relationship.

9

The Mother and her Baby

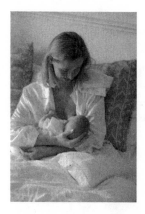

THE CLOSENESS OF MOTHER AND BABY

The mother naturally reaches out her arms to hold her baby. As soon as possible she likes to feel him close to her, nestling in the crook of her arm with his head on her breast. She gazes with wonder and awe; can anything so perfect be born from her? This tiny, firm being has been cradled in her body for so long – she has known the child and yet not known him; they have learned together, both in pregnancy and in labour, the subtle rhythms of each other's bodies – and he was so indissolubly part of her that she was unable to recognise him as a person distinct from herself. However fiercely possessive the mother may be in the first weeks after birth – and there is often a passionate tenderness in the way in which she wants to protect her child – the separation of the umbilical cord heralds the beginning of a new existence, an individual life.

It is only because they are now distinct and separate beings and the baby is no longer rocked in the darkness of her body that the reciprocal relationship of love and need is possible and finds its fullest expression in the experience of breastfeeding. The baby begins to establish a relationship with the world through his mother. 'In the instinct to make contact (first by touch and then by visual "touch" of another being) the inborn *Thou* is very soon brought to its full powers, so that the instinct ever more clearly turns out to mean mutual relation, "tenderness." '[1] The first experiences of love and caring for another are given the baby in these times at the breast.

From the child's point of view birth may have come as a surprise, but we have little evidence to confirm that it is always traumatic and that it gives rise to the first anxiety, which forms a pattern for all later reactions to threat, as Otto Rank asserted. But if this is true, the child who has been born naturally and easily is obviously at an advantage. A newborn baby can have no conceptual understanding of its journey down the birth canal, but probably it is in a state of great neurological excitation. Its nervous system is suddenly flooded with stimuli. Though it used to be thought that the baby was born into what must be 'a big, booming, buzzing confusion',[2] we now know that the undrugged newborn who is in a quiet, alert state, as is usual for some forty-five minutes after birth, is learning about the environment and sending out signals to which, if we are attentive, we can respond. The first 'conversations' are initiated by the baby, and before we can begin to understand interaction between the mother and her baby we need to appreciate the spontaneous and orderly sequences of behaviour that are characteristic of the healthy newborn. Our task is to synchronise with these.

If the birth has been easy it is remarkable how soon the baby stops crying when the mother holds her, how soon the wail of protest is stilled, and with what willingness, as if returning to the breast rather than finding it for the first time, the child suckles in the safe haven of her arms.

The woman who is able to relax while holding her baby – and above all when feeding – lets peace and contentment flow into her, and is less likely to have difficulties in the feeding

---

[1] Martin Buber, *I and Thou* (trans. Ronald Gregor Smith), T. and T. Clark, 1937.

[2] William James, *Principles of Psychology*, New York, 1890.

relationship than one who cannot relax. Relaxation is just as important after the baby comes as it was before.

SOME DIFFICULTIES

Sometimes if the birth has been long and difficult, or the baby is premature with a nervous system not yet sufficiently mature to cope with the world, or has been doped with opiates which the mother received during labour, she starts off at a disadvantage, and feeding is no delight.

Whenever possible, the baby should remain with the mother, for her to give the love that is welling up in her and to fondle and stroke him as all babies should be fondled and stroked. Unless there are very serious and important reasons why mother and child should be separated, and prematurity is not necessarily one of these, she should be free to create in those early days the close relationship of love and need which is the basis for all personality development. She will probably face difficulties in the feeding relationship; the baby may be apathetic and not want to feed, but she has a chance to know and observe her baby in a way that she can never do with one who is isolated in a hospital nursery. If she does not feel that in the space of ten or twenty minutes she has to get a certain amount of milk into the baby, which is what often happens when babies are brought to their mothers only at feeding times, she will not give way to despair. A baby who does not want to suck just then can suck later, and perhaps would prefer a number of small feeds to four or five large ones.

A good way of getting an apparently unresponsive baby to turn towards the breast and to grope for the nipple is gently and lightly to stroke the child's cheek nearest the breast. A baby always turns towards a stroking movement at the side of the mouth. It does no good at all to push the baby's face towards the nipple, to open its mouth forcibly, to put glycerine or honey on the nipple or on the baby's tongue, or to squirt milk into its mouth.

Whilst slapping a baby, tickling his feet or jogging him up and down may wake him up at least temporarily, these activities are not likely to increase his appetite. The over-active, crying baby who seems to fight the breast, can be cocooned in a shawl and held firmly and calmly, but it is unlikely that battening his arms down, fixing his head in a vice-like grip, and holding him as firmly encased as an Egyptian mummy, will add to his content. An over-excited baby is best fed when still half asleep and certainly before he has had time to cry himself into a state of panic. Sometimes these babies are best lifted from the cot or pram still on the mattress, so that they are handled as little as possible before a feed. They may also like to be fed in a darkened room or, at any rate, away from bright lights. The mother may find herself rocking as she feeds or singing softly, a spontaneous response to the need for a peaceful atmosphere. Each mother will learn for herself what is best for her baby.

Babies are not frightened by their arms waving in front of their faces, as some people believe. In fact, they very soon get rather interested in them and discover them as playthings, so this is also no reason for swaddling a baby into a solid, immobile bundle. Some babies scratch their faces badly, and the answer to that is to cut their fingernails rather than to tie their arms down.

You may be concerned about the way in which your newborn baby snuffles, squeaks and sneezes, and lie awake that first night listening to noises and strange types of breathing which you feel sure are not natural. Although this can be alarming, unless the baby is grunting with each breath taken, it is quite normal. A sneeze is a convenient way of clearing the nasal passages and young babies tend to sneeze a good deal.

You may worry also about little sores on the baby's skin. The baby should either be oiled or washed carefully and patted completely dry in all the creases of its body, especially in the area of the buttocks, behind the ears, in the folds of the neck, arms and legs, and between the fingers. A little cream can be smoothed on after the bath, but the skin must be dry before this is done or there will soon be caked lumps of grease in the creases. Cream will also become sticky and unpleasant if the baby is allowed to get overheated or to cry until she is hot.

Bathe your baby in a leisurely way in a very warm room. Then there is no need to rush and handle the baby hastily, and both can enjoy the process. *Everything should be prepared and at hand in advance* and you should be able to sit comfortably. Little actual cleaning of the baby can be done when in the bath as you must concentrate on holding the slippery bundle. So the buttocks should be washed with an unscented soap and the folds and creases of the skin washed gently with small cotton wool swabs whilst he is lying on a big towel on your lap before going into the water – eyes and face first, buttocks last, and a fresh swab for each area. The hair can be done next when necessary, by holding the baby's head over the bowl of water with the body wrapped up in the towel, using a small bowl of fresh water for rinsing.

Cotton wool should not be left in contact with the buttocks, as it tends to cling and also to overheat the baby.

The hair should be brushed with a firm brush with rounded bristle ends – not a very soft baby brush.

Beyond this there is very little that you need know about care of a new baby, for now the essential needs are food and love. So this chapter concentrates on breastfeeding and the intricacies and problems of the feeding relationship.

SUCCESSFUL BREASTFEEDING

Most of us with first babies are unprepared for the responsibilities of motherhood. Girl children may be given little or no preparation, except through doll play, for motherhood. And even their dolls are babies no longer, but teenagers with jutting breasts and elaborately back-combed hair styles. In our modern two- or three-child family, children share very little in the care of younger siblings, and it is accepted that babycare is limited to the mother of the child, much of it taking place in privacy. It is still rare to see a mother breastfeeding her child openly.

It seems incredible that some people could think of breast-feeding as indecent, but women are sometimes forced to sit in toilets in restaurants and other public places in order to perform the simple, natural act of feeding a baby. A first-time mother of thirty told me that she had never seen a mother feeding her baby except once in West Africa. She covered a breastfeeding photograph exhibition I had organised for her newspaper and there saw for the first time a white woman casually putting her baby to her breast. When she had her own baby she said, 'Please be more evangelical and encourage women to breastfeed in as many places as possible and to be unabashed about letting people see. It would be a public service to all future mothers.' But not all mothers have the courage or confidence to breastfeed openly in this spirited way. Girls are still leaving school, even after courses in childcare, without ever having seen a mother breastfeeding, and with no knowledge about it, and boys are even more ignorant about breastfeeding, a central element of mothering without which the human race would never have survived.

The single most important thing to remember about breastfeeding is that nearly always *supply equals demand.* You cannot save up milk for the baby by putting off a breastfeed. If you want more milk you have to feed more often, and if your milk is in short supply a feed every two hours, for a period of anything up to twenty-four hours, will almost certainly produce fountains of milk. This simple rule is easily forgotten, especially when you are doubtful about whether you can breastfeed or are confused by contradictory advice.

Breastfeeding can be quite painful during the first ten days or so, and no woman need be distressed if it proves not to be an unalloyed pleasure.

One of the difficulties that you may encounter in the early days is breast engorgement. Although painful *it is a good omen for successful breastfeeding.*

If you become engorged when the milk first comes in, any time after the first twenty-four hours, you can suffer intense pain. The breasts fill up and become hot, tight and enormous. Rope-like knots stick out on the side of your breast under your arms, and the nipples recede under the surrounding inflamed mass so that the baby cannot get a grip on them. He must be able to get not only the nipple into his mouth, but also part of the areola (the brown area surrounding the nipple).

If you have expressed colostrum occasionally during the later months of pregnancy you will be able to express a little milk to ease the discomfort *immediately* you notice this. It is important to be able to do it yourself, as it may occur in the middle of the night when no midwife is available to help you. Anyway, many women do not like their breasts being treated as simply milk-producing machines and do not want them touched by helpers if it can be avoided.

Holding the breast with one hand cupped under it, rhythmically press with the thumb and first finger of the other hand just above and just below the areola, and *think of the milk flowing*. Soon large drops of milk will begin to ooze out into the cup or washbasin. As you see it you begin to feel what seems like a great rush of milk from higher up in the *other* breast – the 'let-down' reflex – and a steady stream will pour out from the breast you are 'milking', bringing tremendous relief. Stimulation from milking results in the release of oxytocic hormone from the posterior pituitary. This contracts the smooth muscle fibres of the small milk ducts, so forcing the milk into the big ducts, from whence it emerges through the nipple. You will probably not need to continue rhythmically pressing, as simple pressure on the breast will be sufficient for it to stream out in a great arc.

If you are unable to start the flow by expression in this way, you may need to massage the breast a little first. Holding one hand cupped under the breast, rub firmly with the palm of the other from side to side on the upper side of the breast. Then try expressing again. If still nothing happens and you are very uncomfortable, you can gently squeeze hot water over your breasts. Lean over a washbasin or bowl and, dipping a sponge into water as hot as you can comfortably bear, pour water over and along the outside margin of the engorged breasts until milk drips steadily. You can keep the milk flowing with steady pressure of the fingers of one hand, whilst supporting the breast with the other, until you are comfortable. Stop then, as over-expression will stimulate the breast to produce still more milk. If even this fails, a breast pump will relieve you. You can hire one from a breastfeeding counsellor, buy one at the chemist's, or may be able to get hold of one if you ring your midwife.

If your nipples feel sore, keep them well oiled or creamed so that they remain supple; and go back to nature and sunbathe them. Tell the midwife or doctor if the discomfort persists longer than a day. If your nipples are allowed to dry in the air or in the heat of the bulb from the bedside lamp before replacing your bra, you can probably avoid any soreness during the first weeks of feeding the baby.

If your breasts leak, and most women experience some leaking in at least the first six weeks or so, wear an absorbent pad inside the bra over the nipple. This is shaped to the curve of the breast. Leaking from the breasts does not mean that you have too much milk. Washable tops are best, and you will need to change your underclothes and bath frequently, or you soon smell like a cheese market. Gifts of good soap, aromatherapy bath oils and non-allergenic body lotions and creams are greatly welcomed by the nursing mother. A too tight bra or top will press on the breasts so that, as they fill up towards feed times, milk may pour out. It is also necessary to change sheets and pillow-cases frequently, as when you are asleep your breasts may be pressing on the bed. In the days after the milk first comes in it may help to put an old towel underneath the top half of your body.

You may wake early in the morning with your breasts very full and tender. If the baby is asleep, express some of the milk, and you may be able to get to sleep again for a little while. This problem occurs not only in the first weeks but when the baby first decides to sleep through the night. However, the milk supply will soon adjust to this.

Some Lactation Rituals of Doubtful Value

Niles Newton, writing of the differences between markedly successful and unsuccessful breastfeeding, says:[3]

'Successful breastfeeding is the type of feeding that is practised by the vast majority of mothers all over the world. It is a simple, easy process. When the baby is hungry, it is simply given

---

[3] *Maternal Emotions*, Hoeber, USA, 1955.

a breast to suck. There is an abundance of milk, and the milk supply naturally adjusts itself to the child's growth and intake of other foods. It never occurs to the mother to worry about whether the baby is getting enough. The milk is ready and waiting to satisfy the baby's needs. Both mother and baby enjoy the process so much that weaning tends to be postponed rather than hastened.

'Unsuccessful breastfeeding is a type of breastfeeding that is typical of the modern American urban mother. This type of breastfeeding is a difficult and tenuous process. There is constant worry about whether there is enough milk for the baby. The mother is expected to regulate her diet, her sleep, and her habits of living to help make her milk good and plentiful. She worries about washing her nipples, and about which breast to give, and when and how long to give it. She often weighs the baby before and after feeding to see whether the baby has got enough, and is advised to express the milk remaining in her breast by hand after each feeding – a laborious process. Often the supply of milk is so insufficient that bottles must be resorted to to supplement the breast milk. Breast abscesses and engorgement, and nipple fissures and erosions frequently cause extreme pain. The pain, the work, and the worry of unsuccessful breastfeeding make early weaning part of the unsuccessful breastfeeding pattern.'

It is for reasons like these that we need to reassess the value of the lactation rituals in our culture and see whether, in fact, they are helping or hindering us in the feeding relationship.

Breastmilk is not only a nutritious food. It is a living fluid, adapted to each baby's needs. Your milk is just right for your particular baby. It has been discovered that mothers of very pre-term babies secrete milk especially rich in growth factors compared with full-term milk. Babies who suckle energetically and get lashings of milk receive a lower solute milk that satisfies thirst without making them overweight. Babies who suckle more languidly and drop off the breast as soon as they get interested in something else obtain a richer milk that satisfies hunger.

If you have a good milk supply do not make efforts to empty

the breasts, or even one breast, with each feed. It may be a practical impossibility, as the milk continues to flow, and if you change over breasts you feel the let-down reflex again in the other. So 'complete emptying of the breasts' either by the baby alone, or by the baby and expression by hand afterwards, is not necessary and is only useful if you want to stimulate an inadequate milk supply.

One of the most dangerous of the doctrines is that even though a mother is feeding 'on demand', each breastfeed should be regulated by the clock – the baby should have so many minutes at one breast, and then be whipped over to the other side for so many further minutes, when the feeding experience is abruptly terminated, the baby burped, cleaned up, changed, and put down till next time.

Where both mother and baby love feeding times and have pleasure in their relationship with each other, breastfeeding is not an isolated act reserved for set times of the day for a predetermined number of minutes. The child is not a car the tank of which has to be filled with petrol. Nor is it a dangerous animal or little tyrant, gnawing at her nipples and draining away her strength.

All a newborn baby's sensations are centred in the mouth, in the groping sensitive lips and tongue.

> 'My Palate is a Touch-Stone fit
> To taste how Good Thou art.'[4]

To separate a baby from its mother is to tear the child away from the source of life. He needs to feel his mother's loving care as she cuddles him and warms him with her body, strokes his limbs and tiny fingers and the fine down on his cheeks, and as she responds to his quest for the sweet milk it is her privilege to give him.

It is terrible for both the mother and her child to be deprived of these early satisfactions in their relationship – no less real for the mother than for her baby.

---

[4] Thomas Traherne, 'The Estate', *Poetical Works*, Dobell, 1906.

There may be health benefits for the mother, too. Women who do not breastfeed are at greater risk of breast cancer.

The woman reaches out to know her baby. The basis of all the confidence she has in herself as a mother is laid then. She wants to be able quietly and in her own time, without interference, to feel her way towards her child. She begins to learn that it is not enough just to love her baby; she must let her *know* by her warm bodily presence, flesh to flesh contact and her answer to her need for cuddling and for milk, that she loves her. What does she like? What doesn't she like? Often the mother wants to be completely alone when she feeds so that she can experiment a little without feeling that she is likely to be criticised for her clumsiness of movement. She patiently observes her baby and discovers how she likes to be held and whether she minds her reading at the same time or wants her whole attention. She shifts position so as to get more comfortable herself. Occasionally someone sitting quietly watching her feeding her baby can suggest certain changes in handling which can make it much easier and pleasanter for both. But it is not the midwife's task to take businesslike command of the feeding situation, to put the nipple into the baby's mouth and hold her there, however desperately she wants to, however much she feels she could do it all so much better herself.

Breast and Bottle-feeding

The relationship of the child at the breast with his mother is not simply that of feeding, of getting nourishment – as any mother knows. But books on babycare, apart from an approving reference to the psychological benefits to the baby which are supposed to be derived from breastfeeding, rarely go into detail about the nature of the relationship, or about the psychological effects on the mother.

We are told on the one hand that breastfeeding is important and desirable, and that it is our duty to feed our babies ourselves if we possibly can because breastmilk is sterile, is just right for the baby, is at the correct temperature, and gives him the comfort of our arms and our complete attention, and, on the other hand, that it does not matter a bit if we cannot feed our babies ourselves because modern methods of artificial baby feeding – in the hands of an intelligent mother – are sterile and hygienic.

But of course breasts, fortunately, do not feel like bottles, and the communication of emotion by muscular tensions, the plasticity of the nipple, the flow of milk, and other involuntary physical means is possible only when a baby is breastfed. This is the great advantage that breastfeeding can have over artificial feeding, but conversely it obviously has disadvantages in a mother who is under stress, or for one reason or another feels that she cannot *give* milk to the baby.

One reason why some women dislike breastfeeding is that they feel that it – and childbirth too – is something 'primitive', too elemental an experience for a civilised woman to be expected to enjoy. Breastfeeding makes such a woman feel like 'a peasant' or 'a cow', degraded to an almost animal level of existence. There are great cultural variations. Just after my first child was born, a French minister at a diplomatic dinner called across the table to me, 'And have you much milk for the baby?' – an unheard-of thing in Britain, which would have been positively shocking in the USA at that time, where in many hospitals women used to be given routine injections before birth in order to inhibit lactation. The wording of some books giving advice on infant feeding does not always help; the reader is instructed to try and become cow-like – a particularly unfortunate simile when the woman, who may well have endured what she considers a humiliating experience during pregnancy and in the birth, is longing to be her former self again. You do not need to be particularly sensitive to dislike being compared to a cow. As we might expect, however, this feeling is rare among women who have found joy rather than degradation in birth. But where revulsion exists and is strongly felt it should be a contraindication to breastfeeding, for this relationship is a personal matter, and if a woman struggles to do it because she feels she ought to, she is likely to run into many difficulties. If she could relax and enjoy feeding with a bottle it would seem the obvious solution. It is her loving touch that her baby needs, and unsuccessful breastfeeding can be a very frustrating and disturbing experience for both mother and baby. Breastfeeding is the best sort of feeding there is. But unsuccessful breastfeeding comes a poor second to happy bottle-feeding.

To some mothers breastfeeding is almost an erotic experience. In *The Second Sex* Simone de Beauvoir compared heterosexual sex unfavourably with breastfeeding: 'The fusion sought in masculine arms – no sooner granted than withdrawn – is realised by the mother when she feels her child heavy within her or when she clasps it to her swelling breasts . . . The infant satisfies that aggressive eroticism which is not fully satisfied in the male embrace.' Many women take delight in the feeling of the child at the breast and speak openly of the intense pleasure it gives them. Breastfeeding – like sexual excitement – encourages uterine contractions, and hence, the rapid involution of the uterus to its non-pregnant state. Often mothers notice more severe 'after-pains' in the days following birth when the baby is nursing. Women who have these contractions are more likely to be successful with breastfeeding than those who do not have them. Others recognise the erotic element in breastfeeding and dislike it intensely. They do not wish to confuse what for them are two distinct levels of experience, the sexual and the maternal, and breastfeeding may be unpleasant for this reason. Some women cannot feel sexual delight from stimulation of their breasts while they are still feeding their babies. If they do not realise that this is quite a normal feeling they may get a little frightened. They may wonder whether childbirth has ruined their sex life. GPs do not as a rule mention this subject in the brief discussions they have with their patients; midwives tend to find it embarrassing and irrelevant, and it is probably not a subject which a woman feels is serious enough to go to an 'authority' for advice. Some men take delight in seeing a woman breastfeeding and feel no resentment of the ten or eleven o'clock breastfeed at night. But others cannot help feeling a little jealous of the baby then.

This is certainly not a contraindication to breastfeeding; it simply means that some adjustments are necessary.

We have seen that the child does not come to the breast only for food. Her mother's arms form the centre of the universe. She is the giver and sustainer of life and from her touch comes all comfort and joy. It is tragic when a mother treats her child as an enemy, an invader who comes to suck her dry and tire her out and take away her youth and attractiveness, leaving her weary and worn, only to scream and rage for more after a few hours and batten on to her again like a leech. There is a John Bratby painting of a self-sacrificing Madonna in a state of complete physical exhaustion in an untidy kitchen cluttered with tins of baby food and other ritual implements for feeding a large, fat, muscular baby who is the Son whom she worships, the adored child before whom she lays her life. Some conscientious mothers feel they are locked in a struggle with the baby and are advised to 'show the baby who is master', 'Let him see you are in command.' But these are extraordinary words to use about this most tender and subtle of human relationships.

A Baby at the Breast Learns to Trust Life

'The amount of trust derived from earliest infantile experience does not seem to depend on absolute quantities of food or demonstrations of love, but rather on the quality of the maternal relationship. Mothers create a sense of trust in their children by . . . sensitive care of the baby's individual needs and a firm sense of personal trustworthiness within the trusted framework of their culture's lifestyle. This forms the basis in the child for a sense of identity which will later combine a sense of being "all right", of being oneself, and of becoming what other people trust one will become.'[5]

Ian Suttie[6] saw the anxiety, hate and aggression which Freud believed to be primary instincts, and the drive for power which Adler believed to be a characteristic of human nature, as the pathological results of the refusal of the mother to give to her child, or her withdrawal from the child who still needed her, her absence leading to terrifying loneliness. Aggression, he

---

[5] Erik Erikson, *Childhood and Society*, Penguin 1975.
[6] *The Origins of Love and Hate*, Kegan Paul, 1935.

claimed, was not a spontaneous emotion; it was a result of rejection by the mother or fear of that rejection by the child. The good mother is the responsive mother, the mother who is *there* when the child needs her, the mother who does not deny her feelings of tenderness. 'Our adult, grudging, materialistic minds have decided that the baby gets the best of the partnership with the mother, and we talk of the mother's "sacrifice". The mother–child relationship however (to the child's mind) is a true, "balanced", symbiosis; and the *need to give* is as vital, therefore, as the *need to get*.'

Play at the Breast

One of the most important experiences the child at the breast can have is that of *play*. However rushed a woman is, and however efficient she considers herself, she should realise that the baby is not there just to suck like a machine. First of all, the child plays only with lips and tongue, and only later learns the pleasure of stroking her breast or T-shirt with his fingers and the palm of his hand, or of 'bouncing' or bumping her breast, or even pounding, and enjoying its elasticity and texture.

At first a baby's keenest delights are in the area of the mouth and from the first weeks of pleasurable sucking she may try licking, pecking, rolling the nipple between her lips, nibbling and making small plosive movements of the lips against the sides of the breast if she is allowed to nestle in and play with her mother's body. There is nothing wrong with this, even though midwives tend to frown on this playing at feeding and fear that the mother will end up with painfully sore nipples. The baby who makes nipples sore is the one who battens on to the breast without getting a good mouthful, urgently hungry and clamouring – and chewing on the nipple stem, not the one who can casually play whenever she feels like it and who feels the closeness of her mother's flesh when hunger is satisfied.

Planning your Day

To achieve this relationship with your baby it is easiest if you can organise your day around the baby, rather than struggling to fit in the baby with a set routine. This means putting off going back to work until as late as possible in the first year. Many women do not have any choice about this. But if you do have flexibility, the baby should come first. Hard as this sounds, once you have a relaxed attitude to housework – and to activities outside the home, too – it is easier to evolve a routine which fits in approximately with the baby's needs. A newborn baby has a pattern of sleeping, eating and nuzzling play of which you have to become aware before you can guess roughly the most convenient times to get supper in the oven, do the supermarket trip or get on with your thesis, or crash out. It is the mother who is fighting her baby and getting more and more tense while she listens to the screaming, who finds the greatest difficulty in finding time to do things. In dealing with a tiny baby, the easiest way is to omit 'shoulds' from our thinking and enjoy the baby just as he is.

Human beings are more important than the dirty laundry and unwashed dishes. It does not really matter what other people think, though it raises your spirits if you can keep one room clean and tidy. Just for once, get in convenience foods and ready meals. It's worth shopping around ahead of time and checking labels to find those that are healthiest. (Actually, maybe 'just for once' isn't that accurate. Anyone with a baby, especially if there are other children as well, needs to be able to grab something from the freezer when you have had a glut of salads and there is no time to cook. There is nothing immoral about this!)

Even a baby's physical health can be as, or more, dependent upon tender loving care than on hygienic surroundings. In the classic study by René Spitz,[7] out of ninety-one babies in a foundling home who were given every physical attention, their diet carefully planned, and whom 'no person whose

---

[7] 'Anaclitic Depression', *The Psychoanalytic Study of the Child*, Vol. II, International Universities Press, 1946.

clothes and hands were not sterilised' could approach, but who were deprived of maternal love, thirty-four died, and most of the rest were severely retarded. In the control group of children left with their unwed mothers the babies developed normally, and not one died.

It is easiest for you to like each other if you feed 'on demand'. Gradually you will see that the baby can bear to wait a little for food, and can adjust the feeds a bit to suit your convenience. No baby should be left to scream with rage and fright; small babies are not 'naughty' when they cry. They are either in pain or frightened or frustrated. To a newborn the universe is still totally unorganised and shadowy. After some weeks she begins to trace a pattern and expect definite activities. When you pick her up and cradle her in your arms in the way she knows, she is going to be fed. When she hears the water rushing and smells the comfortable scent of towels airing, it is going to be bathtime. Gradually she begins to appreciate the security of an approximately mapped day.

We can imagine that to the new baby hunger is a terrifying experience. Not only is it painful, but she has no knowledge that the torture will ever cease. Adults smile with amused tolerance as her wail rises in a crescendo of fury, but those who imaginatively relive this experience of early babyhood will not smile. For the child is in terror. She knows nothing but desire. She feels completely isolated and lost.

Books on babycare, getting the child weighed regularly, test weighing before and after feeds, cannot tell a mother when her baby is hungry. Only the baby herself can do that. *Before the child begins to learn from the mother, the mother must learn from the baby.*

'Topping-up'

If you decide to give a top-up feed because the baby is not gaining any weight the milk can be prepared before giving the breastfeed and offered afterwards in a bottle, a narrow-rimmed cup, or even a wine glass. The baby can suck it from a spoon, too. The best way of topping up is to express some breastmilk after a feed when you know you have plenty of milk – usually the early morning one – and keep it in the fridge to top up an evening feed. The more feeds of commercial baby milk you give, the more your breastmilk supply will be reduced.

So if it isn't essential to top up with artificial milk, steer clear of it. Forget about 'follow-on' milks, too. Continue breastfeeding instead. Baby food manufacturers try to persuade us that our babies need their products, and to undermine breastfeeding. The World Health Organisation has called for the banning of all breastmilk substitutes, but multinational corporations are evading this. The global market for baby milks and foods is US$ 17 billion and this is rising by 12 per cent every year. The UK has one of the lowest breastfeeding rates in Europe.

It is unlikely that a baby requires extra drinking water, even in hot weather.

It is not necessary to drink excessive quantities of liquid when breastfeeding. Drink just as much as you want. Many women feel thirsty as the milk flows, and like to drink at the same time as the baby. If it is a hot drink be ready for the first time the baby lashes out with a fist when you least expect it and knocks the cup over. Once a baby is kicking and waving her arms around it is unwise ever to drink hot liquid with her in your arms, or allow anyone else to do so.

Encouraging your Milk Supply

The more stimulation the breasts are given by the baby's sucking the more likely are they to respond by producing milk. A hungry baby wants to be fed more often, and in this way the supply is soon increased. Demand regulates supply quite naturally.

Sometimes milk ducts get blocked and you notice a red patch on your breast. The treatment for this is to ensure that the baby is well latched on to the nipple and areola, with a good mouthful of breast. Relax and enjoy long feeds so that the baby can unblock the duct by suckling energetically. Cupping the breast in one hand, massage it with the other, gradually freeing the milk ducts while the baby sucks. Use your thumb to massage towards the nipple. If you develop any inflammation an old remedy, and one that works, is to tuck a cold cabbage leaf inside your bra. Wash some large cabbage leaves and keep them in a plastic bag or box in the coldest part of the fridge.

It is not necessary to have a single clock in the house to breastfeed a baby. There is no need to look at the time or work out how long he has gone between feeds or note down how many times you have fed in the last twenty-four hours, even though you will be constantly asked. Timing breastfeeds is dangerous, because the mother has her eye on the watch instead of the baby, and is not concentrating on giving the milk and the pleasure of its flow as she might be if she were not so uncertain of herself and lacking in confidence. Shift the baby over from one breast to the other side when the rate of swallow to suck slows down, i.e. when the baby has to press the breast more often before swallowing a mouthful, or begins to look around and get interested in other things. You do not need to observe this consciously; you just feel it is time to change over, and react to the change of rhythm. Then you let him go on at the second breast as long as he wants. When he begins to play around, spend a little longer enjoying him, letting him play with the breast, and then change him.

Whilst a baby still minds waiting for food it is best to change her after feeds, or at any rate after she has had one side, rather than before, and also better to bath after a feed if you can do it without bouncing her about too much and making her sick. Babies vary greatly in the ease with which they bring back food, but you can help by learning the technique of undressing, bathing and dressing the baby again without unnecessary movements. Ideally, you should only have to turn the baby over once when undressing, but this rather depends on the sort of clothing. It is useful to have neck openings wide enough for clothes to be slipped on over the legs, or cross-over or envelope neck openings.

Life with a new baby is life in the fast lane! To get the rest you need make a habit of feeding the baby on a bed or couch with your feet up, making yourself really comfortable and luxurious if possible, with a rug and a hot water bottle if you are cold, a drink and a book.

When things seem to be getting on top of you – and at times they are bound to – drop everything as soon as you can and take to bed for a rest. Ten minutes of relaxation and peace then is better than hours of it later when you feel weary and ill. But this is easier said than done – especially if you have other children!

TONING MUSCLES

The midwife will give you a list of exercises to do. If you are in hospital the physiotherapist will come round to teach you suitable exercises for the puerperium (the six weeks following childbirth). These are usually started the day after birth, and are graduated to exercise muscles without straining them.

One of the most important exercises is to tense the muscles of the pelvic floor. If you have had stitches you will not be able to do this at first as it will be painful, but do it as soon as it does not hurt. It is important to consider this not only as an exercise for set times of the day – though to ensure that you do not forget it, it is a good idea to do it every time you feed the baby and whenever you are on the phone – but to cultivate a habit of holding these muscles firm.

YOUR DIET

During the puerperium many women find they get constipated. If you are up and moving around and doing postnatal exercises which massage the abdomen, often all that is necessary is to have raw fruit, plenty of fibre, including porridge and wholemeal bread, and if you wish, laxative foods such as stewed prunes or figs. All straining on the lavatory should be avoided.

It is not necessary to eat large quantities of protein in the form of meat and fish in order to feed a baby. Many vegetarians find no difficulty in breastfeeding.[8]

---

[8] I am a vegetarian, and breastfed my twins for nine and a half months without strain or deterioration in health.

NURSERY MATTERS

You are bound to be given good advice by nearly everyone you come into contact with – friends, relations, people at the supermarket check-out, the health visitor, nurses at the clinic, your mother, and in books, magazines and newspaper articles. Advice coming from professionals may be as contradictory as that from casual acquaintances. For a woman who has just had her first baby this is especially confusing in the first few weeks. If you struggle to try all the things that are recommended you will lose self-confidence. Some of these ideas may be odd. I remember when I had my first baby offering her 'pip-and-peel water', which a baby book advised contained essential nutrients. It entailed boiling apple pips and peel and straining the mixture. Common sense took over after a few days of this and I just breastfed her. Though all this advice that pours in is irritating, it is a sign of people's love for babies. If you realise this you can take even the most officious of instructions with good grace.

The baby must be allowed to cry and the mother must get some rest, she will be told, for if the child does not cry 'his lungs won't expand'. But a woman is rarely able to rest while her baby is crying, and should not try to. If she wants to lie down she can take him with her into bed. The baby's lungs will expand all right anyway.

She must eat certain foods she heartily dislikes or her milk will go. Unless the baby wears woollen booties, bonnet and gloves she may be told that he is cold, and people will worriedly feel his hands and feet. He ought to be weighed, given gripe water, extra vitamins, iron supplements, magnesia, water between feeds, cereal – all these and other suggestions may be made.

Your baby is an individual. Whatever advice you get, remember that babies are different, and that they have personalities, even from the beginning of life. Bear in mind, too, that however many baby books you have studied, *the baby has not read them.*

The simpler the baby's clothes, the better. The easiest baby clothes have all the openings either at the front or back so that dressing and undressing are simple. Long strings and ties are best avoided as the baby soon starts sucking these. Unless it is windy a baby is unlikely to require a hat. Booties always get kicked off and lost as soon as the baby is moving at all, and mittens stop him from exploring his fingers. They will also get sucked and very dirty.

Vest, nappy, open-leg style plastic pants, baby-gro and coat should be sufficient, with warm shawls or blankets for snuggling in. As soon as she begins to kick it helps to have capacious baby bags.

To feel if a baby is warm enough, touch the back of the neck, which should feel comfortably warm. If you are not sure, feel her tummy and back.

You don't need a lot of special baby equipment or furniture. Your baby doesn't care if she is wearing a designer bobble-hat or hand-me-downs, and won't know whether she is sitting in a trendy car seat or one you have borrowed from a friend whose baby has out-grown it. Have it checked over to ensure that it is structurally sound.

Put the baby down to sleep on her back. Research shows that babies breathe most easily in this position, so it is safer than lying a baby on her front. If you have your baby in bed with you, don't put a pillow under the baby, and keep the bedclothes loose. Obviously, don't take the baby into bed if you have drunk too much alcohol or are drugged. Research into how mothers and babies sleep together shows that they naturally adapt to each other and move out of each other's way when they sleep close.

Your baby will probably sleep best cuddled up against you, and that is easiest if you have a sling or pouch so that you 'wear' your baby for at least some time during the day. Babies enjoy being rocked, bounced and swayed as you move around. You can even have a pouch that you can tuck under a big shirt so that the baby is in skin contact with you. You can breastfeed with the baby still inside your clothing. In Japan some women wear a special loose coat with a baby pouch inside it in winter.

Weighing can be of little help to you or the baby, and time

is better spent cuddling and playing. Only if the baby is not thriving (or if you think he may not be) is there some point to it.

A breastfed baby under six months does not need any extras. After that age he will enjoy exploring different tastes. It is the mother who feels very uncertain of herself and that she cannot possibly be producing good milk for her baby who starts stuffing him with other things.

If you enjoy feeding and the baby enjoys it, trust your feelings and go on as long as you want. Just remember to introduce new tastes gradually and be laid back about anything that he does not like. Think of weaning as introducing new flavours rather than cutting out breastmilk, and you will find that there will be no abrupt transition, and no weaning 'crisis'. Many people treat weaning as taking something *away* from the baby that he still wants, but it is rather a question of *enlarging the child's experience*. When he likes other foods he will enjoy having them before the breastfeed and then will tend to take less of your milk after. Until that time, it is best to breastfeed first and give a taste or two of finely grated apple or cereal or what you will after he has satisfied his immediate hunger.

There is no need for a baby to have a bottle at all. But if you want to leave him in the care of someone else it is helpful if a baby is accustomed to the idea of milk coming in a bottle in case of emergency. Babies very soon get interested in what their mothers are eating and drinking and enjoy bits and pieces off her plate and sips from a cup.

Cutting out a breastfeed entirely will mean that the milk supply will become less, not more, so if you want to continue breastfeeding, give your baby some breastmilk with each feed.

Despite theory to the contrary, experience has taught some mothers that protest at weaning is not inevitable. It is possible to allow a baby to wean himself. The prerequisite is that you represent the world as an exciting place and that meals are fun for you both. It may help if you eat at the same time. There is no magic about the baby turning nine months which means that you must drop the last breastfeed just then. Many babies enjoy sucking for months, or years, after that, especially at bedtime, and some are ready to drop it earlier.

AN EVOLVING RELATIONSHIP

As a baby gets older he will be able to wait for a feed without becoming desperate, and enjoy filling in the time watching branches of trees in the wind, leaves fluttering, grasses shaking, shadows moving, people passing, curtains at the window or washing on the line. From the moment of birth the mother and baby have begun to grow away from each other, and now a second landmark is reached. The child no longer needs his mother so insistently and urgently; he starts to turn towards the world and its wonders. However strong mother love is and however possessive in the first weeks of the child's life, the relationship must evolve. I have stressed the closeness of the mother-child relationship. It is a living, growing relationship, and its richest reward is found in fruition in adult independence. The child cannot remain bound to the mother. The mother must know when to draw the child towards her and when to let go, and this involves a delicate sense of timing, not only during adolescence, but even in the first months of life.

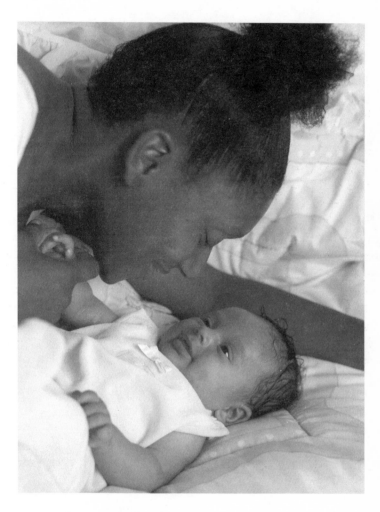

The strength of feeling a woman experiences as a
mother often comes as a surprise.

IO

The Parents' Adjustment

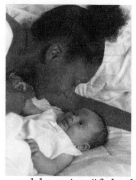

Psychologically, the months after the birth of the first child are a time in which great adjustments are necessary. The mother – even though she hesitates to admit it – may harbour some resentment against the baby who has deprived her of her freedom. Now money may be short and it is difficult to squeeze out enough for clothes, running a car, going on holiday, personal luxuries (if she has any) and presents. She struggles with tasks for which she has not been trained and that recur day after day with monotonous regularity. She feels she is going nowhere – fast.

The baby, too, will almost certainly prove exasperating at times, and even when he is still tiny and she thinks she 'should' be having only sweet and loving feelings about him, she may be shocked to discover that she hates him as well as loving him.

DISAPPOINTMENT WITH THE BABY

It is not easy to admit that you are disappointed in the baby, whom you imagined would be very different and altogether more like your mental picture of an 'ideal' baby.

You are bombarded with baby books, advertisements and

photographs of babies glowing with health and merriment, taken from just the angle at which they look their most roguish and charming. You look at your own baby, who probably has a rash on his cheek, a sore behind his ear, a receding chin, a blister on his lips from hard sucking, eyes that do not yet focus on anything, and skin that seems very pale beside that of these rosy-cheeked babies. What have you produced, you wonder? You feel guilty – first because you must be a bad mother because your child doesn't look like the pin-up babies, and secondly because you feel awful at preferring the look of the advertisement baby to the real live one in your arms. Other mothers visit you with their babies, weeks or months older, who have survived these rashes, sores and other disfigurements and are usually extremely attractive, intelligent and bonny. These mothers rarely mention that their children, too, looked very much like that when they were three weeks old.

Hard as it is, try to relax, and enjoy your baby for what he is, just as he is, at this stage of his young life. That is the beginning of knowing and loving your baby *as a person*. Tell the health visitor any of your worries. But above all, accept the baby's individuality. In a few weeks' time your baby will look much more like the magazine advertisements.

We struggle to be good mothers and know that we are not. Remember, though, that you do not have to be a perfect mother. A 'good enough' mother is just right for a baby. You do not have to be a super-mum.

Being under stress may make breastfeeding difficult. It is easy to get anxious and concentrate all the resources of your mind on a task which is essentially one of instinctive mothering. There may be conflicting emotions, too. You do not want to feel so tied to the baby. You want your breasts to be your own and not belong to the baby.

Perhaps you worry that you do not love your baby, this strange little animal in whom you have a detached but pro-tective interest. Bonding often takes time. It isn't always an instant emotional glue. As you get to know your baby you will discover that you have fallen in love after all, even without realising it.

A PARTNER WHO SHARES

Dick-Read taught that new mothers should be careful to give extra time and tenderness to their husbands after the baby came. Only a man could write that! It was a prescription for behaviour that meant that a woman landed up not with just one baby, but two. The transition to motherhood is difficult enough without demanding that a woman has to mother her partner, too. Yes, the transition to fatherhood can be difficult, and fathers need more support than they usually get, but that cannot be assigned to a new mother as an extra duty she must take on.

A man should be alert to give all the practical help he can and be ready to learn new skills. He ought to grasp the opportunity of paternity leave. In the UK this is now statutory for two weeks after the baby's birth, and you can take one or two weeks in a row (not odd days). This also applies to same sex partners. You need to have worked for your employer for twenty-six weeks by the fifteenth week before the estimated date of birth.

Parents of young children have the right to request flexible work; different or reduced working hours should be given serious consideration. You can find out about your rights if you visit www.maternityalliance.org.uk.

A father or a woman partner should back up the mother in all that she is trying to do, and may need to be a buffer between her and criticism coming from other people. If you start criticising her and make her feel a failure, caring for the baby will degenerate into a series of wearisome chores.

SEX AFTER THE BABY COMES

After the baby is born, a couple can make love whenever they feel drawn together, but it is wise to wait for complete intercourse until there is no more blood-stained discharge. It is normal for this to last from about five days when the involution of the uterus is very rapid to about three weeks in cases when it is taking place more slowly. Often the discharge appears to have stopped, but you notice it again on getting up in the morning or after breastfeeding the baby.

To some women erotic excitement does not return very quickly after childbirth, especially if they feel sore or tender as a result of the birth. Although it is possible for a woman who has had a natural birth to want intercourse three or four days afterwards, it is often at least ten to fourteen days or longer before desire is aroused. A woman wants to be told that she is still lovely and that her naked body can still excite her partner. She does not want to be just a maternal figure, and may fear sometimes that she has bartered the romantic side of their love for the privilege of children, and for becoming a sort of fertility symbol, a goddess of abundance.

She wants to be assured that youth is not suddenly incalculably far behind her. If it is her first child, and especially if it was conceived early in the relationship, she wants to feel that their love has not changed. It does change, of course, and can be richer and fuller as the years go by, but the change can be very difficult to accept. She would rather find again the love she knew than be expected to adapt herself to a love which, though it may be more mature, lacks eroticism, the shock of discovery, and the thrill of a touch which reveals hidden emotions and new desires.

A couple passionately in love with each other cannot believe that their love will ever change or, if it does, are convinced that this must be to something lukewarm, and altogether inferior.

> 'That time when all is over, and
> Hand never flinches, brushing hand;
> And blood lies quiet, for all you're near;
> And it's but spoken words we hear,
> Where trumpets sang; when the mere skies
> Are stranger and nobler than your eyes;
> And flesh is flesh, was flame before;
> And infinite hungers leap no more

In the chance swaying of your dress;
And love has changed to kindliness.'[1]

A woman may find for a time after the baby is born that she is slower to become aroused. So that a couple can share in the same rhythm of mounting excitement, a man should hold back and not allow himself to ejaculate until he can tell from her breathing, and the rhythmic muscular movements inside her vagina, that she is sharing the same crescendo of desire and can reach orgasm.

If a woman has had a tear or an episiotomy which required stitching even light touch of her vagina and perineum may be painful at first, and she is unlikely to want sex until the repair has healed completely. This is as true in a lesbian relationship as it is in a heterosexual one.

When a couple try tentative lovemaking after injury to the perineum, they will probably feel that it is a hopeless failure. She may try to hide the fact that she has not enjoyed it. It is important to be frank about this, because there are things they can do about it.

The stitching is usually at the back of the vagina and is slanted backwards and sideways and out towards the buttocks, or in the mid-line between the vagina and anus. Forceful pressure on the lower edge of the vagina, which at first feels knobbly, rather stiff, and tender, will cause pain. If a couple want intercourse, any pressure should be well forward on the upper ends of the inner lips and on the base of the clitoris. The more a woman is nervous that she will have pain, the more important it is to enjoy prolonged and tender love-play and stimulation of the erogenous zones. A warm bath with a few tablespoonfuls of ordinary cooking salt dissolved in the water before going to bed may help. Her breasts are very sensitive to touch, and all pressure on them should be carefully avoided, as they may be tender and full, and stimulation results in leaking of milk. A partner should concentrate on delicate clitoral stimulation.

---

[1] Rupert Brooke, 'Kindliness', *Collected Poems*, Sidgwick and Jackson, 1923.

If a man is unsure about the exact slant which will be comfortable for his partner, she can help him. She can press the penis further forward automatically by pressing her buttocks together, and this may be easier if her hips are raised on a pillow.

Sometimes a woman notices that she no longer has the lubrication in her vagina which she normally has when sexually excited – lubrication which probably increased during pregnancy – and that her vagina is dry and taut. This makes entry, and any movement inside her, difficult and painful. A lubricant or contraceptive cream will help, or a little almond or some other kind of vegetable oil. The natural lubrication from Bartholin's glands will return later.

As with pregnancy, so with the puerperium, the face-to-face position for sex – with the partner lying on top of the woman – can be very uncomfortable. If both enjoy this, but she finds the pressure on her breasts too much, the partner can kneel with a leg on either side of her body. Some couples are happier with a side-to-side position, or with the lower half of the woman's body lying on top of and across the partner's hips, which has the advantage of freeing her from all pressure and allowing her complete freedom of movement.

Doctors may mention contraception at the examination six weeks or longer after the baby's birth. By then the interior structures should have returned fully to normal. But babies can be conceived within this time, though odds are, especially if a woman is breastfeeding, that ovulation will not start till later, and sometimes it does not return for several months, or until breastfeeding is completed. If a man uses a condom during this time, it is very important that he sees that she is well lubricated, and that he has some more lubricant on the condom itself before attempting entry, as the contact between dry and tender tissues and latex can be painful.

Some women are rather tired after the birth of the baby, as well as a good many months later, when they are no longer the subject of solicitous enquiry from friends and relations, and when they may be trying to run a home, hold down a job, care for a baby, and even entertain. A tired woman cannot be so keenly aware of sexual pleasure as a refreshed and rested one, and all she wants to do when she goes to bed is to drop off to sleep. If the man wants their sex life to improve the best thing he can do is to take some of the work off her shoulders.

CONCEPTS OF PARENTHOOD

For both a man and a woman the experience of birth may have been difficult, in different ways. The woman may be experiencing post-traumatic stress after a birth in which she was denied all choice and control over what happened. A partner may experience similar stress after having to stand by and watch what was being done to her, unable to help. It is easier for him to retreat from his feelings by flinging himself into work, having important appointments, spending time with his pals, or just watching TV. This is what may happen when a man has made no real commitment to fathering his newborn child, or feels disempowered when he tries to help but does it all wrong.

The main responsibility usually remains with the woman. She is the one with the breasts. She is often expected to know what to do by instinct, and may herself expect to know how to care for her baby, exactly how to respond to a bout of crying, for instance, and how to soothe her child and lull her to sleep, simply because she is a woman. If she trusts herself and her spontaneous responses this is largely true. But in another sense mothering has to be *learned*. It is not all instinctive. It is patterned by culture, and each society has its own ways of nurturing babies and rearing children.

There is no denying that the task with which a mother is confronted is demanding. Most women feel, at some time, that they have more than they can cope with. John Bowlby, in his article on 'Psycho-Analysis and Child Care'[2] writes: 'Let us not minimise the difficulties to which the necessity of meeting the infant's needs give rise. In days gone by, when higher education was closed to them, there was less conflict between the claims of

---

[2] 'Psycho-Analysis and Child Care', in *Psycho-Analysis and Contemporary Thought*, ed. John Sutherland, Hogarth Press, 1958.

family and career, though the frustration to able and ambitious women was none the less great . . . let us hope that as time goes on our society, still largely organised to suit men . . . will adjust itself to the needs of women and mothers.'

For some women life is made more difficult than it need be because we bear the burden of an idealised image of the self that is out of touch with the realities with which we have to cope. We suffer under the strain of trying to live up to an impossible ideal of motherhood, which we have gleaned from books on how to bring up babies, baby experts, and the example of our own mothers. It is almost impossible for a woman today, without domestic help, to live up to the standards of housekeeping of fifty years ago. Moreover, standards have changed, not always to be lower but simply different. Nowadays mothers tend to be more concerned that their children develop in a warm, responsive atmosphere where they have opportunities to create and develop new powers over their environment, than they are to see that they are socially presentable, polite and clean, and that they have well-balanced, carefully planned diets packed with all the vitamins and minerals they need, and no fast food.

Some women become very anxious and uncertain of themselves if they have no rule to follow, no strict schedule to guide them. They do not know how to interpret the baby's cries and are anxious that they will be feeding until the baby has colic unless they follow a timetable. If it makes you happier to feed the baby by the clock, do so, allowing some leeway for the baby's hunger either side of the feeding time. That is, be prepared to feed the baby as much as an hour or so early if she is obviously hungry, and leave her undisturbed if she is sleeping when the time for a feed comes round. For, as John Bowlby has said, 'What we must realise . . . is that it is not only what we do, but the way that we do it, which matters. Feeding on self-demand by an anxious and ambivalent mother will probably lead to far more problems than a routine regulated by the clock in the hands of one who is relaxed and happy.'

The old traditions which formed the parent–child relationship have largely crumbled away and – since they no longer possess the validity they once had – we have to replace the custom-dominated sort of relationship, made up of a jigsaw of unquestioned habitual responses and conventional patterns of behaviour, with new perceptiveness about the quality of that relationship and the conditions under which it can flourish. We need to accept the instinctual ground of our being, too, the feelings about our children, the love and the hate that we sometimes have for them, so that we see ourselves and them with honesty. Only under such conditions is it likely that human personality can be given its greatest opportunities of development.

It seems to me that childbirth experienced with joy, in which a couple share, is something valuable not only in itself but as part of the growth of confident parenthood and a positive relationship with our children.

Birth is not merely a mechanical process of getting a baby born. It is part of the ebb and flow of a relationship, and can enrich or deprive it according to how the experience is lived through by both partners.

I hope to have shown in these pages how this experience can bring not only the minimum of pain for the mother, but a deep sense of satisfaction, exhilaration and lasting joy for both parents.

Index